Plant Based Diet

Meal Plan

Beginners Guide for Athletes with 30-Day
High Protein Meal Plan.
Burn Fat Quickly and Increase Strength,
Muscle and Performance!

MANUEL MILLER

INTRODUCTION

Practically speaking, plant-based meals / snacks that could fall within this range would include a few peanut butter sandwiches, a plant-based chili can, a tofu-broccoli stir fry, plant-based meatballs spaghetti, or a plant-based protein shake with bananas and berries. Check out our section on Recipes for a wide range of protein-dense salads, smoothies, and snacks.

Nutrition Isn't Everything Though having enough calories and nutrition is vital to gaining muscle and energy, carbohydrates do play a crucial role in achieving such objectives, because they provide us with the power needed to complete intensive training sessions, while also providing valuable brain control, helping us stay sharp and centered on workouts and competitions.

Evidence has shown that low-carbon diets, including the common high-fat, low-carb ketogenic diet, continue to hinder objectives in training and may delay or even obstruct increases in muscle and power. A new eight-week weight training study in which participants were given the same amount of total calories and protein found That some of those consuming normal carbohydrates managed to gain 2,9 pounds of lean muscle mass whereas those eating low-carbon carbohydrates amassed, ketogenic category acquired zero.

Sacrificing carbs for protein will slow progress, even without going low in carb. A six-month study on rugby players— where calories and fat equaled between two groups — demonstrates that those who eat more plant-based diets with sufficient carbohydrates garnered five pounds of muscle whereas those who eat more protein-based diets instead of carbohydrates gained only one.

The portrayal of the small, thin vegan has become so common that it would be hard for most people to imagine that any person of significant size or power did not eat meat or other animal products. This is because we have been conditioned to believe to build muscle and strength, you also have to eat lots of healthy protein and that protein actually comes from animal feed only.
Of reality, as anyone who has ever seen a (herbivorous) silverback gorilla would quickly deduce, only one of those two assumptions is actually true.

Many people, however, seem to think that humans are more like animals, needing meat or some sort of animal protein to get big and strong at every meal, there are many explanations why this misconception has become so entrenched in popular culture, but the fact is that from the hippie culture of the 1960s to quite recently, many of those who adopted a plant-based diet have been pretty skinny.

This is partially because most people who chose meat / animal-free diets for several decades did so for legal, environmental or health reasons alone, and didn't really care about having big muscles. And those who cared still lacked the basic nutritional understanding required to build plants to feed muscle so energy.

WHERE DO YOU GET YOUR NUTRIENTS FROM AS A VEGAN

Nuts, nuts, beans, fruits and seeds all provide the body with nutritious food, and in conjunction they produce complete protein powerhouses that provide this essential nutrient with ease. Whether it's Multi-Layered Avocado Toast for breakfast, Acadian Black Beans and Rice for dinner, or No-Bake Chocolate Peanut Butter Cookies to please a sweet tooth

Building muscle and strength is really quite simple from a physiological point of view: constantly work out and eat a huge volume of food. If you work out always and eating a few food — or eat plenty of food but don't train enough — whichever one, then you're not likely gaining a lot of muscle or getting much stronger. Whether you eat meat or not this refers to everyone.

To beginner lifters eating "lots of food" means consuming 10-20 percent more calories than the daily maintenance needs and 5-10 percent more for more complex lifts.
The most favorable factor about plant-based food is that it usually produces fewer calories by volume than animal-based foods, allowing us to consume more whole food and feel fuller, without actually adding more body fat.

Those on a plant-based diet need to rely on plant-based foods with a higher caloric content than say, spinach, for those whose top priority is to gain muscle and energy. In fact, this means ensuring that meals and snacks contain heavy amounts of rice, beans, tofu and tempeh, alternatives to meat and dairy, nuts and nut butters, peas, avocados, dried fruits, etc., in addition to fruits and vegetables. Those less obsessed with consuming mostly whole foods may also include plant-based proteins, plant-based protein powders, plant-based protein / energy bars— whatever it takes to get the calorie surplus that is required.

Having Enough Protein: The next important step is to make sure you eat enough protein, because that's what makes up the muscle, and without it you can't build new muscles

Since products such as beef, dairy and eggs usually contain a large amount of protein— while becoming low in other key nutrients such as sugar, vitamin C, folate and potassium — individuals On an animal diet that wishes to build muscle and energy sometimes simply eat more of the foods they're used to, tossing in a protein shake or two for good measure.

Things are a little different for people starting from plant-based diets, in part because "protein" wouldn't be the first ingredient to recall when they imagine "vegetarian" or "vegan" food. More often than not they just think about salad, which includes spinach, onions, cucumber and perhaps some shredded carrots for most people— not exactly a high-protein bowl.

Naturally, in most parts of the world, where meat is not a staple food, there is protein in the form of beans, peas, lentils, tofu, peanuts, other nuts and seeds, etc. However, in so-called "developed" countries, with the exception of peanuts, very few people consume any of the above listed foods daily, and think of plant-based foods as naturally low in protein.

Hence the problem people are constantly bombarded with on a plant-based diet: "Where are you getting your protein from? "Luckily, the plant world is full of protein-rich foods, ensuring that all that people who want to achieve size and strength on a plant-based diet need to do is educate themselves on what ingredients they are and have plenty of them in their daily diet schedule.

There is no scientific basis for the belief that you can not get enough protein from plants, and/or that plant protein sources are "inferior." Which scientific research confirms is how much protein (animal or plant) is required to optimize and/or improve size and strength.

While most people need only eat around 0.8 grams of protein per kilogram of body weight (g / kg) per day— or 0.36 grams per pound (g / lb) — to maintain good health, work based on muscle gain and strength has consistently demonstrated that substantially more protein is required.

Current research indicates that most sports take between 1.2-2.0 g / kg, with endurance athletes at the bottom of the scale, with upper-end bodybuilders and power athletes. If your aim, like professional bodybuilders or powerlifters, is to increase muscle mass and strength as quickly as possible, research shows that as much as 2.2 g / kg can be successful.

It's worth remembering that people who consume a large amount of protein, whether or not they eat animal products, usually rely on protein powders or supplements to reach such higher target numbers. And unsurprisingly, because eating protein at the high end of the spectrum frequently comes at the expense of other nutrients— like carbohydrates— over-focusing on protein can potentially undo progress, as we'll address below.

Since the bodies and aspirations of all are different, the only way to determine what works best for you is always personal exploration.

Doing the numbers Since most people looking to gain more weight and energy are not experienced bodybuilders or powerlifters, we have chosen a range between 1.6-1.8 g / kg (0.73-0.82 g / lb)— deemed more than enough for most competitors — to provide some sample measurements.

Use your weight in kilograms and subtract by 1.6-1.8, or use your weight by 0.73-0.82 to find out how much protein you need to consume per day to live within this range Of eg, if you weigh

77kg/170lbs, that's equal to 123-139 grams of protein a day.

If you eat five times a day, divide this range by five (three meals plus one afternoon snack and one evening snack) and you now have the average amount of protein you need each time you eat. In this case, the 25-28 grams are 123-139 grams divided by five. You can of course quite often eat more protein at one bite of food, and less at another, because your actual daily intake is what matters most.

Recent research suggests that the intake of carbohydrates within a range of 5-7g / kg — or 2.3-3.2 g / lb — is efficient for optimizing gains. Then take your weight in kilograms and multiply by 5-7, or take your weight in pounds and multiply by 2.3-3.2 to measure how many carbs you need per day to help height and strength improvements, Link to Getting and Staying Lean for more on carbohydrates, including the role that unrefined carbohydrates such as bananas, oats, and sweet potatoes may play in getting / staying lean.

Additional Advantages Because plants are filled with many other important nutrients— including starch, healthy fats, vitamins, minerals, enzymes and phytochemicals— a diet based around them can also aid in other ways to build, preserve and defend new tissues, because illustrated in The Plant-Based Advantage.
Some of these benefits include: Increased energy, giving us the motivation and endurance we need to get into the gym and push through tough workouts.
Increased blood flow, which not only provides more oxygen to muscles, but also carries more of the nutrients needed to prevent and cure injuries.
Reduced inflammation: This can serve to speed up exercise

recovery times. Reducing unnecessary inflammation can also improve healing from injuries, taking you back to exercise so much faster.

Increased muscle capacity, which helps us to pull out more reps. One test investigating the impact of eating plant rich in nitrate found that participants were able to bench press 19 per cent more total weight.

As epitomized by the body builders and power athletes — including world-record keeping Strongman Patrik Baboumian, American record-holding Olympic weightlifter Kendrick Farris, and Tennessee Titans defensive line — it was not only important to establish and retain strength and power on a plant-based basis; but rapidly becoming another new reality across a wide range of sports.

CHAPTER ONE
IMPORTANCE AND STRENGTHS OF A PLANT-BASED DIET ALSO IN SPORT

Plant based diets play an important role in cardiovascular health which is important for athletes with stamina. But even well-trained athletes are at risk for heart disease, the review finds. A 2017 study found that there were coronary plaques in 44 per cent of middle-aged and older distance riders or athletes. A low-fat, vegetarian diet is the most scientifically proven successful nutritional method for removing the plaque. A plant-based diet also tackles other main atherosclerosis factors including dyslipidemia, increased blood pressure, increased body weight and diabetes.

Because a plant-based diet usually has a high carbohydrate content, it can also give performance benefits. Carbohydrates are the primary source of energy during aerobic exercise, and a high intake of carbohydrates enhances stamina. But a 2016 Ironman triathlete study found that less than half registered meeting the recommended intake of carbohydrates for athletes exercising 1-3 hours in 24 hours.

Furthermore, the researchers believe that a plant-based diet enhances athletic performance and growth by increasing blood flow and tissue oxygenation and decreasing oxidative stress and inflammation. A diverse intake of citrus, vegetables, nuts, and legumes along with an added vitamin B12 an endurance athlete with all the necessary nutrients including protein, calcium, and

iron needs.
In these metabolic aspects, athletes can benefit by adopting a plant-based diet:

- Reduces body fat and encourages leaner body composition.
- Increases carbohydrates in cereals, legumes, and root crops to enhance glycogen content in muscle cells and increase endurance.
- Increased blood flow to body tissues and oxygen.
- Reduces oxidative damage in fruits and vegetables that are high in antioxidants by fighting free radicals.

HOW MUCH PROTEIN DO WE NEED

How many grams of protein do we need in a day? For a woman it's 0.5 to 1 gram per pound that you weigh. It varies between studies, but this range appears in most. Luckily, it's not hard to acquire. So a 130-pound woman needs 65 grams of protein in a day to maintain a balanced diet.

If she is trying to build muscle, then she should aim for 130 grams per day.
A man's protein intake should be 0.8 to 1.5 grams per pound that he weighs. So a 175-pound man should get 140 grams, and 263 grams if he is trying to really bulk up. Bodybuilders and pro athletes often add protein supplements on top of protein-rich diets. While some protein powders are meat- or dairy-based, vegans only use protein powders that are dairy free (such as pea protein).

It's better for your body to process a divided amount of protein throughout the day instead of all at once. So, for instance, a seitan burger plus a protein shake in one sitting isn't going to provide you with the actual protein contained in those foods. Your body will process whatever you feed it, but it will not always do so optimally. The ballpark amount of protein that your body will use at one time is 30 grams. It takes a couple of hours for your body to process that protein. This is the rhythm in which we usually eat anyway, so getting enough protein is pretty much a no-brainer.

If you're bodybuilding or an athlete, then you need to check your own numbers, because you would require more than usual for meals and snacking. A scoop of protein powder once or twice a day is an easy way to make sure you've added the extra protein you need without stuffing yourself.
As always, drink plenty of water.

Seitan, Tofu, and Tempeh!
Seitan, tofu, and tempeh are protein powerhouses of the vegan world the small quantity of it mean a lot protein and satisfaction. All three products start with vegetables or grains and have been used by cooks for hundreds of years. You can recreate most of your childhood favorites and cherished comfort foods by using one of these ingredients.

Let's Talk Seitan
Seitan is a plant-based product that is made from grains and vegetables. The result of this combination is a textured product that can be sliced, diced, pulsed, and chopped. You can even shape it before cooking into any form, including nuggets or patties. It can be tender and it can be chewy. It's all in the mix and kneading.

Seitan can be bought premade or it can be made at home. Store-bought seitan isn't always marked as such, so you need to look at the ingredients. If the first ingredient is vital wheat gluten, then it is seitan. Be on the lookout for additives and preservatives. As always, making your food from scratch is the best way to really know what you're eating.

Since seitan can be easily made at home, and because it also results in a great product, my vote goes to homemade seitan. It all starts with vital wheat gluten, which is a flour that is 70–80 percent protein. You can buy non-GMO versions, so that's another plus. Ingredients are added for flavor, and then all is cooked low and slow.

Not only do you get a great boost of protein with seitan, you also get fabulous texture and flavor added to your recipes. Plus, it's economical. One pound of raw dough turns into about 2 pounds of cooked seitan. Including all ingredients, that is close to only $2.00 for 2 pounds of a delicious textured product that you can slice for sandwiches, cube into casseroles, crumble into tacos, have as a main course, and so much more.

The last chapter of this book is titled "Let's Make Seitan." You'll find multiple recipes with different flavors and cooking methods.

Tofu Is Versatile

Tofu is a tasteless soybean product that's been around almost 2,000 years. True, it didn't appear in our grocery stores until the 1950s, but it had been completely explored a very long time before that. The love of tofu escaped many of us until recent years, but it has finally become a beloved ingredient. Tofu is made in two forms: silken and regular, and it is high in protein, low in cost, and versatile in recipes. Tofu is some darn good stuff.

Silken tofu comes as a silky mass that adds so much to puddings and desserts and even some types of soup. Silken tofu is undrained and unpressed, and it comes in soft, firm, and extra-firm versions. The version is clearly marked on the package. Even extra-firm silken tofu has a creamy texture.

Tofu that is not silken is called regular tofu and is found in the refrigerated section in grocery stores. Regular tofu is best when it is drained and pressed. And if it is marinated, it will take on the flavor of the marinade.
Silken tofu needs to be drained and/or patted dry. Soft block regular tofu needs to be drained, and medium, firm, and extra-firm tofu need to be drained and pressed. All recipes in this book will state which type of tofu you need and how to prepare it.

If tofu is new to you, then a great introduction to this ingredient is scrambled tofu. You can add so many things to scrambled tofu, and it makes for a filling and High protein breakfast with very little effort. Tofu can also be prepared so that the outside is crisp and the inside is soft. For example, see the recipe "Fried dried tofu and peanut sauce". Marinated tofu can add flavor more easily, and marinated tofu revitalizes the dish. In extreme cases, silken tofu can be used to treat high protein such as puddings and shakes.

How to Press Tofu

There are several ways to press tofu. First open the package and drain away the water. Then stack many paper towels on a dinner plate. Place the tofu on the paper towels and add more paper towels on top of the tofu. Put another plate on top of those towels. Now weigh it down with cans or an iron skillet. The paper towels will soak up the liquid as it is being pressed. Alternately, you can buy a tofu press. The one I have lets you slide your tofu between two hard layers and then there are two latch screws that you tighten. Set the press on its side on a plate and let it drain the liquid from the tofu. This takes about 10 to 20 minutes.

Tempeh, A Little Something Extra

Tempeh is also made from soybeans, but it is different from tofu in many ways. Tempeh is made from cooked and fermented soybeans and is very firm but not hard. It has a unique taste but also can be marinated. Tempeh can be sliced extremely thin or cut into small blocks.

Flavored tempeh products are also available in grocery stores. You can try these and see what you think, but if you buy "original" versions of tempeh you can control the seasonings and flavors. Since tempeh is so easy to cut into any form, you can slide it into just about anything.

BENEFITS OF VEGAN DIET

HEALTHY PLANT POWER WITHOUT CHOLESTEROL

Foods with animal ingredients are often unhealthy. This is partly due to the mostly unhealthy preparation, but also due to the composition of animal products. Substances that are problematic to health, such as cholesterol, saturated fatty acids or purines, are increasingly found in animal products, while they are present in much smaller quantities or not at all in plants. In addition, many health-promoting ingredients, such as fiber and phytochemicals, are only ingested through plants.

NO RISK FOODS IN SIGHT

When we attended the food safety training, we learned that food is divided into groups by the Health Department and assessed according to risk. Eggs, meat and fish are considered to be risky foods, and when they are prepared, increased safety requirements must be met. They are more susceptible to contamination. With one exception (sprouts), vegetable foods are not on this list. Your plant based meal prep is therefore longer-lasting and can also do without cooling for much longer.

TIRED OF HEALTHY SECONDARY PLANT SUBSTANCES

There is no doubt that the regular consumption of vegetables and fruits is essential for the implementation of healthy eating. In addition to legumes and whole grains, vegetables and fruits are a rich source of nutrients, including vitamins, trace elements and fiber.

The food groups also contain phytochemicals that influence various metabolic processes. Various health-promoting effects are attributed to secondary plant substances. For example, their mechanisms of action include stimulating the immune system, lowering blood pressure and expanding the blood vessels. In addition, plant substances achieve neurological anti-inflammatory and antibacterial effects.

According to some studies, the regular consumption of vegetables and fruits can reduce the risk of high blood pressure, lower coronary heart disease and stroke. There are also signs that regular fruit and vegetable consumption can prevent weight gain. Perfect conditions to make your meal prep plant based!

ANIMAL PROTEIN VERSUS VEGETABLE PROTEIN

Protein is not the same as protein. Protein, also called protein, is a macronutrient and indispensable for a balanced diet, since the human body cannot produce proteins or amino acids itself. In the past, protein was a synonym for meat and is therefore still associated with many, especially with animal foods.

Nowadays the topic of "proteins" is omnipresent and seems more important than ever. Whether marketed as "protein muesli", "protein bars" or "protein curd", the marketing departments come up with something to sell their products. The days when only bodybuilders talked about protein and amino acids are long gone and more and more people are dealing with both vegetable and animal proteins.

But what's the difference and what does that mean for your meal prep plant based? Vegetable protein sources on average provide more valuable ingredients than animal alternatives. For example, hemp is a rich source of B vitamins, calcium, potassium, iron and magnesium. Generally, all types of legumes provide B vitamins, folate and other minerals such as iron, magnesium and zinc.

COVER NUTRIENTS

It is obvious to most people that eating lots of vegetables and fruits is healthy. However, many are unsure whether it is actually possible to cover all essential nutrients with plant based meal prep. At this point we can clearly say from our own experience: YES! All nutrients, such as iron, calcium, magnesium, can be covered with plants. Only B12 needs to be supplemented! Contrary to many opinions, B12 does not naturally occur in meat.

In animals, B12 is also artificially supplemented. Therefore, the following applies to plant based meal prep: keep an eye on vitamin B12. However, this also applies to people who eat animal products. It is also worth taking a look at vitamin D3 and vitamin K2 (regardless of the diet)! This is related to the year-round light and sun conditions in Western Europe.

But back to plant based meal prep: with a bit of know-how, all nutrients can be covered with plants and if you eat a varied diet, you don't have to worry about whether you are consuming all the nutrients. Another reason to give plant based meal prep a chance in the future!

PRE-PROGRAMMED TASTE EXPLOSION

Your taste buds also benefit from a change in diet! Especially when you start to focus on plant-based food, you will be pleasantly surprised at what the culinary journey has in store for you. Suddenly you discover a variety of otherwise neglected vegetables and fruits, cereals, vegetable milk and nutmegs.

The preparation of plant based dishes often arouses creativity and the spirit of discovery in the kitchen and in the supermarket. Many report that their taste buds become more sensitive after eating and that they taste more intense. We have also had this experience. Through the plant based diet, we have relived the familiar taste.

HEALTHY WITH PLANT-BASED FOODS

Many people find entry into the plant based diet due to health problems. In the case of numerous clinical pictures and complaints, a plant-based diet is recommended by doctors. Cancer patients are often advised to leave out milk products. Heart sufferers are advised not to eat meat.

People with acne or neurodermatitis are also often advised not to eat milk products. A wholesome plant-based diet can also have a positive effect on blood, cholesterol and blood pressure values. If done correctly, the plant based diet and plant based meal prep can relieve symptoms and be used as a preventive measure. Some report having reached their ideal weight and positive effects on their digestion after changing their diet.

IMPROVED SLEEP

Sleep is essential. Good sleep is essential, especially in a busy everyday life. Your body and mind need to regenerate at night and recharge your batteries. Since you cannot need long sleep or not sleep through! At this point, meal prep plant based comes in handy, because: Many types of vegetables and nuts contain vitamin B6, tryptophan and magnesium, which have a positive effect on sleep.

GOODBYE MIDDAY LOW

Animal fats strain the body, especially at warm temperatures, because they have to use a lot of energy to digest them. The digestion of meat takes us so much that we would like to sleep after a hearty roast. This tiredness is known to many as the midday low. If you design your meal prep plant based, you will quickly notice that there are much lower or no lows. So if you are tired of the midday low after your lunch, definitely try to keep your meal prep plant based in the future.

ABILITY TO REGENERATE

Regeneration means "relaxation". The ability to regenerate is understood to mean the potential of humans to recover after physical and psychological stress. For example, a plant based diet can help regulate body weight. The “strength-to-body weight” can be influenced favorably, which improves sporting performance. The high proportion of valuable micronutrients in a balanced plant based diet is another reason why performance and the ability to regenerate can be improved. Another point why you should make your meal prep plant based.

CONSTITUENTS OF DIETS MACRONUTRIENTS

The Carbohydrates: also called carbon carbohydrates, sugars or more commonly, are the primary source of energy. They also contain the fibers, which we will define a little later.

The Fat: fatty acids also called "fat" or fat are molecules that form the organic fat. They play an important role in the constitution of cell membranes, energy production, and body temperature and more generally in the metabolism of the human being.

The Proteins: they are essential molecules for the life of cells and the constitution of human tissues (muscles, hair, skin, etc.).

Macronutrients are molecules that provide energy to our body or that participate directly or indirectly in metabolism. They are called "macro" in order to differentiate them from micronutrients such as vitamins, minerals, enzymes, etc.
Macros is the abbreviation for macronutrients, which refers to carbohydrates, fats and proteins. "They are called macros because we need them in greater amounts than micronutrients, which include vitamins and minerals. Almost everything we eat is made up of macronutrients, and sometimes also micronutrients, which we need in smaller quantities.

Carbohydrates
It is the main source of energy of the body.

As you have guessed, it's about sugars, and yes sugars, we'll always need them. Everything depends then which sugars to privilege, and there, it becomes more complicated.

In theory, these are the complex sugars to favor at the expense of simple sugars, but that does not help you much!

What are the foods based on complex sugars and those based on simple sugars?

Simple sugars have a high glycemic index (Glucose and sucrose ...) they are present in sweets, pastries, classic white sugar, in many prepared dishes, sauces (ketchup, bbq sauce, sweet and sour) Complex sugars, meanwhile, have a low glycemic index; they are present in cereals (whole grains, attention!) and legumes.

Sugar in fruits is also an excellent source of energy, but we must not forget that fructose must first be treated in the liver before 'be used by the body, and it cannot be part of the complex sugars, it is a so-called fast sugar, but does not have a too high glycemic index, (IG: 20 against 100 for glucose), which differentiates it especially glucose classic is that the carbohydrate intake is supplemented with a contribution of fiber, minerals and vitamins.

The Protides

In common parlance we often tend to call them "proteins", but this is an abuse of language, and yes, in fact the protides is a sort of "family" grouping proteins, amino acids, and peptides.

When we talk about proteins "protiderotides" we immediately think of our muscles, and yes you know well they are made up, but we must not forget that they are also made of 70% water, moreover the water content of our body represents on average about 65% of our mass, small parenthesis

Back to our proteins, except the muscles (myosin, actin, myoglobin) , they are also present in our hair, nail our skin (keratin), but also in our red blood cells (globin).

They provide a multitude of functions within the cells:

- Cell renewal

- Role of protection (hair, nails, skin)
- Physiological functioning (information transmission, digestion, immune defense)
- Secondary energy role (after carbohydrates)
- and it is also our only source of nitrogen (essential for life) , and yes it is a present element to link amino acids to each other.
- Proteins are of animal or vegetable origin (legumes, cereals)

Contrary to many received ideas, vegetable proteins are not of less good quality than animal proteins, on the contrary.

Indeed, animal proteins also contain so-called saturated fats (we'll talk about it later), favoring weight gain, cardiovascular risks and clot formation, on the contrary vegetable proteins are rich in fibers without any saturated fat.

Lipids

Despite their demonization, it is a primordial macro nutrient essential to our proper functioning.

Lipids are an important energy store, they are essential to regulate the temperature of our body, and very importantly, they are one of the major constituents of membranes and the nervous system, indeed lipids surround and strengthen our lymph.

On the other hand, lipids are not all of the same quality!

This is where the difference, always and again, good and bad fats, so we distinguish different types of fatty acids: saturated, monounsaturated or polyunsaturated.

The saturated = to limit! They increase the cardiovascular risk as stated above (contained in fatty meats, sausages, butter or cream, vegetable fats biscuits and industrial dishes)
Mono-unsaturated = also called omega-9 contained in oilseeds (almonds, hazelnuts, walnuts ...) and avocado

Poly-unsaturated = these are omega 6 and 3, these are essential fatty acids, our body is unable to synthesize them, they contribute to the proper functioning of our cardiovascular system, some studies have demonstrated that omega-3 fatty acids promote lipolysis (provision of fat to provide energy to the body) it is not beautiful, so do not hesitate to consume virgin oils first cold pressed (olive oil, rapeseed),also in oily fish, but I cannot encourage you to consume since they too often contain heavy metals such as mercury, and especially for our biodiversity and ethics, it is better to leave them there where he is, it was the little ethical parenthesis

An individual's macros are calculated as a percentage of the total calories consumed. "So, for example, if you are an active middle-aged and 60k-weight individual who goes to the gym regularly and follow a 1600-calorie diet, you need 40% of your calories to come from carbohydrates, 30% of proteins and 30% of fats.

These proportions would be normal for those who do not train for a living, or for people who are active, but not for endurance athletes. This is what those calculations would look like:

1600 x 0.40 = 640 calories from carbohydrates

1600 x 0.30 = 480 calories of protein

1600 x 0.30 = 480 calories from fat

"To convert those calories figures into grams, carbohydrates and proteins are divided by 4, because both carbohydrates and proteins provide 4 calories per gram, "and fat by 9, because fat contributes 9 calories. per gram. " This is how those calculations would work:

640/4 = 160 grams of carbohydrates

480/4 = 120 grams of protein

480/9 = 53 grams of fat

The proportion of macros will change according to your objectives. "It is important to take into account your level of activity and the type of exercises you do,

For example, if you are strength training you will need to increase your protein intake to facilitate muscle recovery and prevent injuries. While if you focus more on cardio, you will have to increase carbohydrates to prevent the wear of glycogen stores.

WHAT IS THE EASIEST WAY TO CALCULATE YOUR OWN MACROS?

When entering your data in an online macro calculator: age, height, weight, sex, activity level, target weight, frequency and intensity with which you lift weights. If It Fits Your Macros, which also asks when you want to achieve your goals, or Healthy Eater, which is simpler, but produces similar calculations.

MICRO AND MACRO NUTRIENTS

Nutrients can be divided into two categories: macronutrients and micronutrients. Macronutrients are nutrients that the body needs in large quantities. These provide energy (calories) to the body. Micronutrients are nutrients that the body needs in smaller amounts. Click the links below to discover the various nutrient functions your body needs, recommended dietary intakes, and food sources.

MACRONUTRIENT

- carbohydrate
- protein
- fat

CARBOHYDRATE

Role in the body

- Fuel during high intensity exercise
- Spare protein (to maintain muscle mass during exercise)
- Central nervous system fuel (your brain!)

Recommended allowance

Sedentary individuals: 40-50% of total calories a day must be carbohydrate

Regular exercise: 60% of total calories a day must be carbohydrate

Athletes or those involved in intense training: 70% of total calories a day must be carbs (3.5-4.5 grams of carbs per pound of body weight).

Note: 1 gram of carbs = 4 calories

FOOD SOURCE

- Grains (choose almost whole grains for additional benefits)

- Dairy products (most often choose low or no fat)
- Fruit (more often to select whole fruit than fruit juice)

PROTEIN

ROLE IN THE BODY

- Tissue structure (organ tissue, muscle, hair, skin, nails, bones, tendons, ligaments and parts of plasma)
- Part of the cell plasma membrane
- Involved in metabolism, transport, and hormonal system
- Make enzymes that regulate metabolism
- Involved in acid / base balance to maintain a neutral environment in our body

Recommended daily allowance

Sedentary individuals: 0.36 grams of protein per pound of body weight

Recreational activities: 0.45-0.68 grams of protein per pound of body weight

Athlete: 0.54 to 0.82 grams of protein per pound of body weight

Teen athletes: 0.82-0.91 grams of protein per pound of body weight

Bodybuilders: 0.64-0.91 grams of protein per pound of body weight

For calorie restriction: 0364-0.91 grams protein per pound weight

Maximum amount of protein available to the body: 0.91 grams of protein per pound of body weight

Note: 1 gram of protein = 4 calories

FOOD SOURCE

- Legumes (beans)
- lentil

- Soy products such as tofu
- Peanuts and nuts
- Whole grains (quinoa, oats, brown rice)
- seed
- Meat replacement products
- Some vegetables

FAT

ROLE IN THE BODY

- Energy reserve
- Protect important organs
- Insulation
- Transport of fat-soluble vitamins

Recommended allowance

20-35% of total calories a day should come from fat

Less than 10% of total calories a day must be obtained from saturated fats (coconut and plum kernel oil, shortenings, butter, cream , full fat dairy products)

Note: 1 gram of fat = 9 calories

FOOD SOURCE

- oil
- nuts
- seed

MICRONUTRIENTS

- Water-soluble vitamin
- Vitamin B1

- Vitamin B2
- Vitamin B6
- Vitamin B12
- Vitamin C
- Folic acid
- Fat-soluble vitamins
- Vitamin A
- Vitamin D
- Vitamin E
- Vitamin K
- mineral
- calcium
- potassium
- sodium
- iron
- zinc
- water

VITAMIN B1: THIAMINE
FUNCTION

- Needed to release food energy
- Prevents beriberi

FOOD SOURCE

- Whole grain
- Dried beans
- beans
- Peanuts

VITAMIN B2: RIBOFLAVIN
FUNCTION

- Necessary for building and maintaining body tissue

FOOD SOURCE

- Whole grain
- Green and yellow vegetables

VITAMIN B6: PYRIDOXINE

FUNCTION

- Helps develop the nervous system
- Involved in blood production
- Helps break down protein and glucose to produce energy in the body

FOOD SOURCE

- Potato
- Chickpeas
- Yeast
- Nuts
- Bulgur
- Banana

B12: COBALAMIN

FUNCTION

- Promotes proper growth and development of the nervous system

FOOD SOURCE

- Reinforced cereal
- Nutritional yeast

- Algae

VITAMIN C: ASCORBIC ACID
FUNCTION

- Helps growth hormone formation
- Needed to build strong gums, teeth and bones
- Antioxidant

FOOD SOURCE

- Citrus fruit
- cabbage
- Berries
- pepper
- Folic acid

FUNCTION

- Supports DNA and protein construction
- Helps maintain the intestinal tract
- Bone growth aid
- Prevent birth defects in the nervous system

FOOD SOURCE

- Dark green leafy vegetables
- yeast
- Wheat germm

VITAMIN A: RETINA
FUNCTION

- vision
- Healthy skin

- Healthy hair

FOOD SOURCE

- The body can make vitamin A from vegetables that contain carotene
- carrot
- sweet potato
- Other red orange vegetables

VITAMIN D

FUNCTION

- Promotes strong teeth and bones
- Prevent rickets

FOOD SOURCE

- mushroom
- Dairy and fortified non-dairy products
- Reinforced cereal
- Cod liver oil
- tuna
- Salmon
- egg yolk
- Produced by the body when exposed to sunlight

VITAMIN E

FUNCTION

- Prevents cell membrane damage
- Protects vitamin A
- Blood production assistance

FOOD SOURCE

- Seeds and nuts
- Vegetable oil

VITAMIN K

FUNCTION

- Aid in blood coagulation
- Food source
- Green leafy vegetables
- Produced by bacteria in the colon

CALCIUM

FUNCTION

- Maintain teeth and bones
- Helps blood clots
- Helps nerve and muscle function

FOOD SOURCE

- Dairy and fortified non-dairy products
- Dark green vegetables
- sardine
- clams
- Oyster
- Legumes
- Almond

POTASSIUM

FUNCTION

- Regulates intracellular water balance
- Helps nerve function
- Important for heart rhythm

FOOD SOURCE

- Orange
- banana
- grain
- potato
- Dried beans

SODIUM

FUNCTION

- Adjust water balance
- Stimulates nerves

FOOD SOURCE

- Table salt
- Bread
- Almost everything

IRON

FUNCTION

- Form blood cells
- Transports oxygen throughout the body

FOOD SOURCE

- Dark green vegetables
- Whole grain
- Whole grains such as brown rice and quinoa
- Legumes
- lentil
- nuts
- seed
- Dried fruit

ZINC

FUNCTION

- Aid in transporting carbon dioxide
- Helps heal wounds
- Form enzymes
- Food source
- Whole grain
- Dairy and fortified non-dairy products
- Legumes

WATER

FUNCTION

- Moisturizes tissues such as mouth, eyes and nose
- Protects body organs and tissues
- Helps prevent constipation
- Dissolves minerals and other nutrients to make them accessible to the body
- Regulate body temperature
- Lubricate joints
- Reduces kidney and liver burden by washing away waste products
- Transport nutrients and oxygen to cells

THE BENEFITS OF COUNTING MACROS

A positive aspect of eating by adjusting to your macros is that each macro performs a unique function. As runners or endurance athletes, it is important to have enough carbohydrates to avoid "crashing into the wall", but you also don't have to be too forgiving.

It's about getting the right amount of each one right, so as not to fall short or exceed your body's needs. By achieving that balance, your body will function at its highest level and you will recover properly. It also activates other systems such as immune, digestive and sleep. "It's like a group of workers in which everyone does their job so that the whole body works at its maximum performance.

It is clear that this "work" depends on your level of activity and your objectives. "If you are an athlete, macros are very important. Also, if you eat adjusting to your macros, you don't have to eliminate any important food groups or deprive yourself of anything.

But if you want to lose fat, gain muscle, it is very important to consider the source and quality of the food you eat. "I have seen people who count macros stuffing themselves with donuts because 'it fits their macros', but they perform less and feel worse than if they had opted for sweet potatoes or other types of carbohydrates," he adds.

THE BAD THING ABOUT COUNTING MACROS

In an IIFYM diet, the important thing is not to deprive yourself of something, but to feed you so that your body functions in the most effective way. But counting macros can take time. Not only do you have to know the proportions, but you also have to measure food on an appropriate scale. So if you feel lazy to weigh everything you eat, counting macros is not made for you.

In addition, monitoring, tracking and weighing everything you eat can create an unhealthy relationship with food. Anytime the numbers go up and you like to control your diet. But if you have suffered eating disorders in the past, counting macros is probably not a good idea.

Like any other diet, counting macros is not a panacea. It can help you make the body function very effectively, and even serve you to reach certain goals, but remember that the most important thing is the quality of what you eat. As an athlete, you know that diet is only part of the equation, so the best is what best suits your lifestyle and, therefore, you manage to maintain in the long term.

HOW TO HAVE MORE ENERGY WITH PLANT BASED DIET

Diet plays an immense role in our rising and falling levels of energy. If we nutritiously feed our bodies with food that stimulates the thyroid gland and supports energy metabolism, we can successfully feel rejuvenated throughout the day, regardless of our sometimes daunting to - do lists.

A diet based on fresh fruits and vegetables, legumes, nuts and seeds, and plants filled with whole grains is a very lively diet to follow. Obviously so because it is great for digestion (a process that uses a lot of energy), can provide rest for a good night, and will help control blood sugar.

The digestive system is needed for energy, growth, and cell repair, but some food products require excessive digestive effort, and are therefore more draining. The animal-based protein is especially hard to digest. Further secretion of the stomach acid, pancreatic enzyme secretion and bile synthesis are needed to break down animal protein because it is more acidic. It means greater intestinal complexity, and the need for digestive capacity.

On the other hand, plant-based protein is much easier to digest, and does not contribute pressure to your digestive system. Naturally occurring plant foods are also packed with complex carbohydrates that play an important part in the metabolism of energy.
When you eat a diet based on plants, you will often get a better night's rest in the process.

This is because more foods rich in vitamin B6, such as bananas, sweet potatoes, squash, walnuts, lettuce, broccoli, avocados, and peanut butter will most likely be included. Vitamin B6 is important for rest and relaxation, as it helps to regulate activity in the nervous system. If you get a good night's rest, the next day you will undoubtedly have more energy.
In fact, a plant-based diet is perfect for controlling blood sugar levels, which will help you stay energized regularly by stopping a jump and then dropping in blood sugar.

ANABOLIC BOOSTING FOODS

It doesn't matter if you are looking to increase your testosterone level so you can have a better quality of life, better performance between the sheets, better muscle mass, or athletic purposes, you can't deny the fact that there isn't any solution that will be as effective as using anabolic steroids.
You can get results that will place you above most of the human population with totally natural sources of steroids. This is great

news since these sources won't have any side effects. These are extremely for you.

The Body's Natural Steroids

If you hear anybody talking about raising the amount of anabolic hormones in their body, they are normally talking about their testosterone levels. This is the main sex hormone in men, and it can influence the body in large ways. It can help your overall well being, general health, bone mass, and muscle mass.

If you get testosterone from outside sources, your body doesn't have to make its own. Testosterone, just like any other steroid hormone gets synthesized from cholesterol. It is a fact that has been proven that one side effect of taking medicines for reducing cholesterol is that it causes a drop in testosterone.

Testosterone is normally created inside the Leydig cells in men. How much it makes gets regulated by a luteinizing hormone.

There are many vitamins and minerals that can influence how much testosterone gets produced. The important ones are vitamin D, magnesium, and zinc.

Everyone of these has a role in producing testosterone, and a deficiency in just one could cause a disturbance in the process, and this could cause a drop in the levels.

If you tried to make up all these deficiencies with supplements, you would be taking over 100 pills each day. Yes, you could do this, but there isn't any need to. Except for a few exceptions, most of these deficiencies can be fixed by changing up your diet.

Vitamin D3 is the main one that could be a huge problem. It is hard to get enough with food, and if you don't live on a sunny beach, it will be impossible to get enough through exposure to the sun. For this main reason, you need to take a supplement.

Nobody can talk about testosterone without talking about sleep and exercise. Compound, heavy exercises have been known to create an anabolic effect on your body while growth hormone and testosterone get synthesized and then released when you get a good quality of sleep.

When you can combine all this with the food you eat, these are the things you have to do to fix it if you want your testosterone levels really soar.

Let's look at some natural foods that you need to eat if you want to boost your testosterone:

- Celery

Celery has many health benefits. It prevents muscular degeneration and can improve your eye health. It can reduce the pain and swelling in joints. Celery can prevent UTIs in women. It can reduce cholesterol and blood pressure levels. It can improve immunity and prevents cancer. Celery can help you get relief from asthma and migraines. It can promote better cardiovascular health. It can manage the symptoms of diabetes. Celery is a good way to get Vitamin K. If you love green shakes, more than likely you put it in them. If you haven't considered it before, you need to think about it.

First and foremost, celery is high in Vitamin K. This help keep the best levels of testosterone. Just one cup can give you one-quarter of your daily recommended intake.

Androstenol and androstenone are powerful anabolic hormones that are found in celery. Increasing your intake of celery should have a positive impact on your testosterone levels. Since there isn't any potential for side effects, celery can be something worth looking into.

- Wild Oats

Wild oats or Avena sativa is cereal grain that is rich in nutrients. They can increase the luteinizing hormone. When you eat wild oats on a regular basis, it can help lower your blood cholesterol.

Everyone knows that eating oats for breakfast is a good thing. But most don't realize that they provide anabolic effects such as tribulus terrestris. It can also increase the luteinizing hormone levels and frees up testosterone that has been bound to make it more prevalent in the body.

- Figs

Figs can help you manage your weight. If you need to gain some weight, eat them with milk. The leaves of figs can reduce or prevent symptoms for asthmatic people. Figs can prevent the loss of vision that is caused by macular degeneration. Figs can help correct sexual dysfunction. They can reduce the risk of getting colon cancer. Figs can get rid of diarrhea and prevent constipation. They can help strengthen bones and stay away from losing calcium through urine. Figs are potassium-rich, which helps regulate the absorption of sugar in people who are diabetic. Figs can prevent hypertension. Figs can lower cholesterol that puts you at risk for coronary heart disease.

This might just be the tastiest food on this entire list. Figs are a great source of the amino acids arginine and leucine. They also contain Vitamin K, the B Vitamins, potassium, magnesium, iron, and fatty acids.

Arginine can help you produce testosterone. It can also help your blood flow, and that makes it popular with bodybuilders and anyone who wants an extra boost when in the bedroom.

Figs also are high in fiber and pectin. Pectin is a soluble fiber that helps get rid of bad LDL. Figs make a great healthy, and tasty snack.

- Quinoa

Quinoa is a complete source of protein, and this is rare for plant sources. Quinoa can provide all the amino acids including the ten

that our bodies don't produce by itself. Quinoa operates like a grain, but it has a huge protein to carb ratio.
Quinoa provides you with Vitamin E, selenium potassium, Vitamin B6, riboflavin, zinc, thiamine, iron, copper, folate, phosphorus, magnesium, and manganese.
The Andes in South American have given the world powerful food such as maca, with quinoa being no exception.
The main substance in quinoa that makes it so interesting is ecdysteroids. These are a group of compounds that function like androgens or testosterone. These are natural alternatives to steroids. Even though they are full of steroids, humans can consume the, and there are many bodybuilders who do, in fact, use them.
Adding raw, uncooked quinoa to smoothies will give you about one third of your daily zinc, 55 percent of your daily magnesium, and 46 percent of your daily folate. Raw, uncooked quinoa is full of minerals and vitamins.

- Avocado

If you don't love avocados or guacamole, here are some reasons you should.
Other than being full of more than 20 vitamins along with copper, magnesium, and zinc, it is a good source of monounsaturated fatty acids. This is what you need to consume if you would like to boost your testosterone levels.

- Fava Beans

These aren't a common food, but they do contain the strongest natural growth hormone supplement L-dopa.
Just a half a gram of L-dopa can increase the circulation of growth hormones. The highest concentration happens one hour after you have eaten them. Other studies show they can increase luteinizing

hormones and testosterone.

- Asparagus

Asparagus has nutrients such as Vitamin K, Vitamin B6, magnesium, and D-aspartic acid.

If you haven't ever heard about D-aspartic acid, it can increase your testosterone levels in just a short amount of time. It is great for increasing your fertility.

Ancient Greeks back in the second century used asparagus as an aphrodisiac. Now we know why it actually works.

- Bananas

Bananas might not be at the top of the list of foods you normally eat to increase your testosterone levels, but they should be. They contain bromelain enzyme, potassium, and Vitamin Bs. Bromelain enzymes are normally found in pineapples. This is the thing that causes the biting aftertaste. That is actually the enzymes breaking down the tissues in your mouth. Don't worry; the effects are negligible.

In one study with competitive cyclists, just one gram of bromelain enzymes each day can counteract the effects of endurance exercises on testosterone. The level of testosterone can significantly drop if you do a lot of endurance work. By adding bromelain, athletes don't have to worry about any drops in testosterone levels.

If you do endurance exercises for weight loss or sport, eating pineapple, banana, or supplementing with bromelain is just one way to keep the testosterone levels up.

- Spinach

There are many health benefits to eating spinach. It is full of powerful nutrients like Vitamin D, iron, Vitamin A, and folate. Just like all other leafy greens, spinach gives you calcium, magnesium, and fiber.

Spinach can help strengthen your eyes. It provides anti-aging properties. It is full of omega-3 fatty acids. Spinach contains niacin, folate, riboflavin, Vitamin B1, and Vitamin B6. Spinach is very high in iron. It can help maintain a low blood sugar, prevents constipation, and helps with digestion. Spinach can help your body fight stroke, cardiovascular disease, and atherosclerosis. It can fight wrinkles, acne, and psoriasis. Spinach can lower your blood pressure. Spinach can alkalize your body.

If you know who Popeye is, you know he used spinach's power to get his strength. It doesn't work like that in real life, but it does have extremely high levels of magnesium that has shown to increase testosterone levels.

One study researched how effective a magnesium supplement was on sedentary men and athletes. It found that both had an increase in their testosterone levels. The increase was higher in athletes. It looks like exercise and magnesium are a wonderful combination to help boost your testosterone levels.

Because one package of spinach contains about half of your daily intake of magnesium, it would be best if you took a supplement or add other foods that give you magnesium into your diet, such as pumpkin seeds orchard.

All-Natural Testosterone Boosters

The time that you need to reorganize your diet along with some adjustments won't be anything when the results you get give you a better quality of life, better libido, an energetic life, and a body that is full of muscles.

This list might seem a bit daunting, and this isn't even a total list of the foods that can have an anabolic effect on your body.

Rather than just thinking this is a cool chapter without doing anything to change your diet, write down some of these foods and find out where you can add them into your normal food habits. Grab a banana to have as a delicious snack at work or school. Have a bowl of oats for breakfast to give you a testosterone and protein boost to your day.

Try not to get hung up on anyone food. The main thing is to make sure you are getting enough water and calories to your normal diet along with adequate sleep and exercise. This will become the basis for your success.

TIPS FOR SHOPPING

When shopping applies: Well-planned is usually already won. Anyone who thinks before, what he wants to cook buys more targeted and provides more variety. Generally good: Buy fresh and seasonal goods as much as possible. It tastes better and is often cheaper.

FRUIT AND VEGETABLES

Season: Buy seasonally. Tomatoes, radishes or strawberries have a long journey in the winter and come mostly from the greenhouse. This is at the expense of taste and vitamin content.

Fresh or frozen: Let withered spinach or yellowish broccoli lie down. When in doubt, frozen vegetables are better. It is processed harvest fresh, the vitamin content is higher and the taste better than long-stored goods. Sometimes the handle to preserve is worthwhile. Example tomatoes: Here come fully ripe fruit in the can.

Mature or immature: Ripe fruits give on finger pressure usually slightly and smell good. Some fruits and vegetables can also be bought immature. Apples, bananas, kiwis or avocados ripen at home.

Appearance: The appearance is often secondary: the shinier the apple, the more likely it has been treated with pesticides. You should also ignore size and commercial classes: Especially small fruits are often big in taste.

Packaged fruit: Should you weigh. For cardboard trays, check that the soil is moist. Then down is slush.

Street stalls. Small greengrocers often offer particularly appetizing greens. But you should intensively brush it at home. Car exhaust and abraded brake pads are deposited.

CHAPTER TWO
30 DAYS PLANT BASED PROTEIN RECIPE PLAN

DAY 1

BREAKFAST: VANILLA BREAKFAST SMOOTHIE
Active time: 10 minutes
Total time: 10 minutes
Yield: 1 serving

Protein: 20 grams per serving

This smoothie is perfect for a plant-based break-breakfast breakfast. Only seven **INGREDIENTS**s are required and can be made in less than 10 minutes.

INGREDIENTS
1 frozen banana, slice
1 cup vanilla almond milk
¼ cup old-fashioned oats
¼Cup raisins
1 tablespoon flax seed
¼Cinnamon tea spoon
3 tablespoons of vanilla protein powder

INSTRUCTIONS
1. Add all ingredients to the blender and blend until very smooth.

LUNCH: LOADED CHICKPEA SALAD SANDWICH
Active Time: 15 minutes
Total Time: 15 minutes
Yield: 8 YIELD

Protein: 21 grams per serving

Here's a complete meal for your whole family. It's a big batch, it's quick to prepare, and it keeps great in the fridge or freezer.

INGREDIENTS

- 2 15-ounce cans chickpeas, drained and rinsed
- 2 15 oz cans of pinto beans, drain, rinse
- 2 tablespoons raw shelled hempseed
- 1 tablespoon vegan mayonnaise (add another tablespoon if you like it better that way)
- 1 tablespoon Dijon mustard (add another tablespoon if desired)
- 2 tablespoons lemon juice (optional)
- ¼ teaspoon garlic powder
- ¼ teaspoon paprika
- ½ teaspoon salt
- ¼ teaspoon ground black pepper
- 16 slices whole wheat bread or sprouted grain bread
- 2 avocados, sliced
- 2 ounces baby spinach

INSTRUCTIONS

1. In a large bowl, add the beans and mash. Leave a bit chunky, not completely mashed. Add the remaining ingredients except the bread, avocado, and spinach. Mix well.

2. Spread on the bread slices. Add the avocado slices and spinach. You can also keep any extra chickpea salad in your fridge for up to 5 days.

DINNER: EMPTY BAKED STICKY RICE USING SEITAN

Active time: 30 minutes
Cook time: 30 minutes
Total time: 1 hour
Yield: 4 YIELD

Protein: 20 grams per serving

This dinner recipe takes off socks. Sweet and spicy sauces can be made quickly and easily. There is also a frying pan option!

INGREDIENTS

- 2 cups jasmine rice
- ½ cup soy sauce or gluten-free puddle
- 4 tablespoons maple syrup
- 4 pieces of garlic, finely chopped
- 2 teaspoons of 5 Chinese spices
- 1/2 teaspoon ginger
- 4 tablespoons white wine or rice vinegar
- 1 pound cremini mushroom, cleanly wiped, or cut into large mushrooms in half
- 1 cup pressure cooker Thai nugget
- ½ cup frozen peas

INSTRUCTIONS

1. Add rice to a large pot of 2 cups of water. Cover and bring to a

boil. Cook on medium heat and cook for about 20 minutes or until water is absorbed.

2. If the fryer does not have a built-in insert, insert it now.

3. Mix soy sauce, maple syrup, garlic, 5 Chinese spices, raw inger and white wine in a small bowl and set aside.

4. Put the mushrooms in the air fryer. If you can set the temperature, set it to 350 ° F. Otherwise, just turn it on. Air fryer temperature is built-in and is always cooked at 338 ° F. Cook for 10 minutes. Open the air fryer and add seitan nuggets. If the fryer does not have a built-in self-stirrer, stir. Pour the liquid mixture and beans from above. Stir for 5 minutes and cook.

5. Add the rice and stir well. Heat for 2 minutes. Take out

Note: If you do not have a fryer, you can make this dish in a frying pan. Pre-cook jasmine rice and set aside. Combine the following six ingredients and save. Apply heat to oil in a big mixing skillet. Add mushrooms and cook over medium high heat for 10 minutes. Pour the liquid mixture into the mushrooms. Add the peas and seitan nuggets and cook for another 5 minutes. Add the cooked rice, stir well and cook.

DAY 2

BREAKFAST: WARM MAPLE PROTEIN OATMEAL

Active time: 5 minutes

Cook time: 30 minutes

Total time: 35 minutes

Yield: 2 YIELD

Protein: 23 grams per serving

Do you keep forgetting oatmeal? Make this recipe and you will never forget it. This oatmeal dish that is healthy, warm and slightly sweet will hum during breakfast.

INGREDIENTS

- 1 cup steel cut oats
- 3 tablespoons of raw tbsp, split
- 3 tablespoons maple syrup
- 2 tsp cinnamon
- 1 tbsp sliver almond
- 1 tablespoon currant

INSTRUCTIONS

1. Boil 4 cups of water in a large pot. Add steel cut oatmeal, 2 tablespoons hemp seed, maple syrup and cinnamon and bring to a boil. Reduce heat, cook for 30 minutes without lids, and stir occasionally.
2. In a bowl, serve with almond sliver, currants and remaining hemp seeds.

LUNCH: SPICED GREEN LENTIL SANDWICH

Active Time: 20 minutes
Cook time: 10 minutes
Total Time: 30 minutes
Yield: 8 YIELD

Protein: 14 grams per serving

Lots of texture and wonderful flavors enhance this spiced-up sandwich. It's one of the best veggie combinations you could ask for.

INGREDIENTS

- 1 cup green lentils
- 1 small potato, to equal about ½ cup mashed potato
- ½ cup chopped onion
- 1 carrot, finely chopped in a processor
- ¾ cup old-fashioned oats
- ½ cup pepitas or sunflower seed kernels
- 1 tablespoon hempseed, toasted in shell
- 1 cup breadcrumbs
- 4 tablespoons tamari
- 1 teaspoon ground ginger
- 1½ teaspoons smoked paprika
- ½ teaspoon salt
- ¼ teaspoon ground black pepper
- 1 tablespoon coconut oil
- 8 sandwich buns

INSTRUCTIONS

1. Place 2 cups water and the lentils in a large saucepan. Cover and bring to a boil. Turn down to low and cook for 20 minutes. Drain off remaining liquid from the lentils, if any. Set the lentils aside.
2. Pierce the potato a couple of times with a sharp knife. Wrap in a damp paper towel. Set in the microwave and cook on high for 4 minutes or until you can pinch the potato easily. Peel the potato and mash well. Set aside.
3. Heat 2 tablespoons water in a skillet over medium-high heat. Add the onion and sauté for 10 minutes. Remove from the heat.
4. Add the lentils, potato, onion, and the remainder of the

ingredients to a large bowl (excluding the oil and the buns). Mix well. Form eight patties to the size of your sandwich buns.
5. Using a frying pan, heat it and fry the lentil patties on each side without crowding.
6. Spread the buns with all your favorite condiments and any other toppings of your choice.
7. You may also freeze extra patties for future meals.

DINNER: KALE WHITE BEAN SOUP
Staying time: 8 hours
Active time: 20 minutes
Cook Time: 2 hours
Total time: 10 hours 20 minutes
Yield: 6 YIELD

Protein: 14 grams per serving

This is a simple and tasty recipe and provides a complete meal. Perfect for any night of the week, Let the beans pickle all night and you're on the way.

INGREDIENTS

- 1 pound navy beans
- 1 tablespoon coconut oil
- Coarse onion cup
- 1 garlic, chopped
- ¼ Cup nutrition yeast
- 1 red pepper diced
- 4 chopped Roman tomatoes
- 2 cups of carrot slices
- 5 cups vegetable soup

- 1 teaspoon Italian seasoning
- 2 teaspoon salt
- 1/2 teaspoon black pepper
- 1 lb of kale, coarsely chopped with stem removed

INSTRUCTIONS

1. Put the beans in a large stock pot and cover with about 3 inches of water. Leave overnight to inflate the beans. If you want a simple way to prepare the beans instead of soaking overnight, cover the beans with 2 inches of water in a stock pot. Cover with lid and bring to a boil. Remove from heat and leave uncovered for 1 hour. Drain the beans in a colander and set aside.
2. Put the oil in the same stock pot and heat over medium heat. Add the onions and fry for about 10-15 minutes until soft and translucent. Put garlic and boil for a minute with stirring. Add 4 cups of water, beans, nutritive yeast, peppers, tomatoes, carrots, soups, Italian seasonings, salt and pepper. Cover and bring to a boil. Start the heat and boil down. Cook for about 1 to 1.5 hours until the beans are soft.
3. Add the kale and two cups of water and simmer for about 12-15 minutes until the kale is soft.

DAY 3

BREAKFAST: STACK OF ENCHILADA CASSEROLE

Active time: 30 minutes
Cook time: 1 hour
Total time: 1 hour 30 minutes
Yield: 4 YIELD

Protein: 14 grams per serving

There is nothing like casserole baking and this smells very good. With two different sauces, along with vegetables and tortillas, this dinner is a quadruple victory.

INGREDIENTS

Filling

- 1 cup of diced yellow pepper
- 1 sweet potato, peeled and cut into bite-sized pieces
- 1 cup diced white onion
- 1 tbsp extra virgin olive oil
- 1 tsp salt, split
- ¼ teaspoon ground black hu pepper
- 1 15 oz black beans, drain, rinse
- 2 oz tempe, fine pulse
- 1 teaspoon cumin
- 1 tsp chili powder
- 2 garlic cloves
- 2 cups of red enchilada sauce purchased at the store
- 6 small corn tortillas

White sauce

- 2 tablespoons butter without dairy
- 3 tablespoons flour
- 1½ cup milk without dairy
- Nutritional yeast 1 tablespoon

INSTRUCTIONS

Filling

1. Preheat oven to 400 ° F.

2. Put the peppers, sweet potatoes and onions on the baking sheet. Sprinkle with oil to make sure all vegetables are coated. Spread on a baking sheet and season with 1/2 teaspoon of salt and pepper. Put in oven and roast for 15 minutes. Remove from the oven, stir and return to the oven for another 15 minutes. Check if the sweet potato can be easily pierced with a fork. If not, stir and cook for another 10 minutes. Remove from oven and set aside. Reduce oven temperature to 350 ° F.

3. Add the roasted vegetables, beans, tempe, cumin, chili powder and garlic to a medium bowl.

4. Spread the ¼ cup enchilada sauce on the bottom of the 8-inch square glass casserole dish.

5. Cut the four tortillas into four. Place four compartments in each corner of the casserole, and turn V toward the corner. Place the whole tortilla in the center. Top with a third of the vegetable mixture and spread evenly over the tortillas. Drizzle an additional 1/4 cup of enchilada sauce. Place another tortilla layer as before. Lay another layer using one third of the vegetable mixture, then add ¼ cup of enchilada sauce. Put another layer of tortilla, then put the rest of the vegetable mixture. Set the rest of the enchilada sauce aside.

White sauce

6. Melt the butter in a medium pot. Stir flour and cook for 1 minute. Add milk and heat over medium to low heat. Add nutritional yeast and continue cooking and stirring until the sauce is thickened and boiled down in about ¼ cups. Remove from heat.

Assembly

7. Pour the remaining enchilada sauce over the casserole and spread evenly. Drizzle the white sauce back and forth on the top, but do not spread. Cover with casserole dish lid or aluminum foil sheet. Bake for 30 minutes.

8. Remove the enchilada casserole from the oven and remove the foil. Sit for 10 minutes, then serve in a square.

LUNCH: CHICKPEA TORTILLA FAJITAS STACK
Active time: 20 minutes
Total time: 20 minutes
Yield: 4 YIELD

Protein: 17 grams per serving

Chickpea tortillas have a crepe-like texture and a good flavor blend. These fajitas stacked in layers of spicy beans and mushrooms are great. Who hate Mexican food?

INGREDIENTS

- Chickpea tortilla
- 1 tbsp chia seed
- 1 cup chickpea flour
- ¼ teaspoon sea salt
- 1/2 teaspoon cumin
- 2 tablespoons extra virgin olive oil

Filling

- 1 tbsp extra virgin olive oil
- ½ cup diced onion
- 1 diced yellow pepper
- 8 oz white mushrooms, diced
- ½Diced tomatoes in cups
- 2 teaspoons of fajita seasoning
- 1/2 teaspoon salt
- ¼ teaspoon ground black hu pepper
- 1 15 oz can focus, drain and rinse beans
- 2 tablespoons of raw
- Salsa for decoration
- Avocado for decoration

INSTRUCTIONS

Chickpea tortilla

1. Mix the ground chia seeds with 3 tablespoons of water. Set aside.
2. Add 1 cup of water, chickpea flour, chia seed mixture, salt, and cumin to a medium bowl.
3. Mix until combined.
4. Add 2 tablespoons of oil to an 8-inch frying pan and set on medium heat.
5. Add the chickpea dough in the cup and tilt the dough into a circular shape like a crepe to cover the bottom of the dough.
6. Cook until golden and turn it over. Cook for another minute and transfer to a plate. Continue until all batter is gone and tortillas are made.

Filling

7. Add the oil to a large skillet and heat over medium heat. Add the onions, peppers and mushrooms and fry for 10-15 minutes or until the onions are translucent. Add tomatoes, fajitas, salt and pepper and cook for 5 minutes. Add beans and hemp seeds. Heat through.

Assembly

8. Stack the chickpea tortilla stack from one tortilla on the plate. Spoon about ½ cup of filling. Add another tortilla and ½ cup of filling and continue until all the filling is gone. Top in tortillas, salsa and avocado, Cut into quarters in the shape of a pie and serve.

DINNER: SLOW COOKER SEITAN BOURGUIGNON

Active time: 30 minutes

Cook Time: 9 hours

Total time: 9 hours 30 minutes

Yield: 4 YIELD

Protein: 34 grams per serving

This dinner is rich in flavors such as mushrooms, carrots and citrus. It is easy to make and you will be amazed by its deep taste.

INGREDIENTS

- 2 tablespoons extra virgin olive oil
- 1 cup diced yellow onion
- 1½ cup sliced carrots
- 2 tablespoons dairy-free butter, split
- 2 garlic cloves
- 2 tablespoons flour
- 2½ cup vegetable soup
- 1 tablespoon liquid smoke
- 2 tablespoons of tomato paste
- 1 cup of good Burgundy wine
- 1 bay leaf
- 1/2 teaspoon time
- 1 tsp salt
- 1 pound mushroom, slice
- 2 cups slow cooker versatile seitan ball, cube

INSTRUCTIONS

1. Apply heat to oil using a big frying pan. Add the onions and carrots and fry for 10-15 minutes or until the onions are translucent. Add 1 tablespoon butter. Put garlic and boil for a minute.
2. Add small flour and stir to coat everything and cook for another minute. Make sure the flour is fully functional and the mixture is not showing any dry flour.
3. Add all ingredients from the frying pan to the slow cooker. ½ Stir with a cup of water, soup, liquid smoke, tomato paste, wine, bay leaf, thyme, and salt. Cook over low heat for 6-8 hours.
4. Approximately one hour before serving, fry the mushrooms in a

large frying pan with one tablespoon of butter for about 10 minutes. Add mushrooms and citrus to the slow cooker and cook for another hour.

5. Serve alone or with noodles, potatoes or rice.

DAY 4

BREAKFAST: DELICIOUS QUINOA BREAKFAST CUP

Active Time: 10 minutes

Cook Time: 40 minutes

Total Time: 50 minutes

Yield: 6 YIELD

Protein: 7 grams per serving

Muffins are a breakfast you can easily eat anytime. It is very nice as you can enjoy them at your leisure.

INGREDIENTS

- ½ 3 tablespoons cup plus quinoa
- 1/2 cup spinach
- Sliced mushroom ½ cup
- 1 cup milk
- ⅓ chickpea flour
- Nutritional yeast 1 tablespoon
- 2 tablespoons of raw
- 1/2 teaspoon salt

INSTRUCTIONS

1. Sift the quinoa and rinse well. In a small pot, add quinoa and two tablespoons of water to one cup. Boil, cover and boil down. Cook for 10-15 minutes or until liquid is absorbed. Remove from heat

and set for 5 minutes with cover attached. Remove the lid and fluff.
2. Preheat oven to 375 ° F.
3. Put the muffin cup of paper in 6 cups of muffin tin.
4. Put the spinach and mushrooms in the food processor and process until finely chopped.
5. Add all ingredients to a large bowl and mix well.
6. Divide the mixture into muffin cups. Bake for 20-25 minutes.

LUNCH: PROTEIN PEANUT BUTTER BALLS
Active Time: 20 minutes
Total Time: 20 minutes
Yield: 24 balls

Protein: 10 grams per serving (2 balls)

Here's an easy and healthy treat that you can pop in your mouth any time of the day. Energy-packed with only six ingredients!
INGREDIENTS

- ½ cup creamy peanut butter
- ½ cup maple syrup
- ½ cup powdered soy milk, non-GMO
- ¼ cup flaxseed meal
- ½ cup coconut flour
- ¼ cup peanuts, chopped fine

INSTRUCTIONS
1. Place the peanut butter and maple syrup in a medium bowl. Mix well. Add the powdered soy milk, flaxseed meal, and coconut flour. Mix well and roll into 24 balls. Lightly roll each ball in the chopped peanuts.
2. Store in the refrigerator for up to 2 weeks.

DINNER: SUPER GREAT POBLANO PEPPER
Active time: 15 minutes
Immersion time: 1 hour
COOK TIME: 45 minutes
Total time: 2 hours

Protein: 17 grams per serving

Four huge roast peppers packed with vegetables and spices. Immediately arrange them in a casserole for an unforgettable southwestern style meal. Cashew nuts can be soaked the night before, so you can jump right into preparation.

INGREDIENTS

- Chili and stuffing
- 4 Poblano peppers
- ¾ Cup quinoa
- 1½ cup vegetable soup
- 1 tablespoon coconut oil
- ½ cup diced onion
- 1 garlic, chopped
- 1 cup black beans, drain, rinse
- Fresh, frozen or canned corn cups
- 1 tippotre pepper of advo sauce, small chopped, 1 tablespoon of advo sauce
- 1 tsp chili powder
- 1/2 teaspoon cumin
- 1/2 teaspoon salt

Cashew sauce

- Soak the cup of raw cashew nuts for 1 hour to overnight and drain
- Nutritional yeast 2 tablespoons
- 1 tablespoon tapioca starch (also called tapioca flour)
- 1/2 teaspoon of garlic

- 1/2 teaspoon onion
- 1 tablespoon lemon juice

INSTRUCTIONS

Chili and stuffing

1. Heat the broiler.
2. Place the peppers on the baking sheet and on the top shelf of the broiler. Turn frequently with tongs to darken all sides. After the peppers have cooled, scrape the darkened skin with a damp paper towel or peel with a pairing knife. Grab the edge of the skin with a knife and peel off. Pepper will be packed, so be careful not to tear the pepper. Perhaps they split naturally in one place, so use it as your opening to get rid of the seeds. Set aside.
3. Position the quinoa in a big pot after rinsing thoroughly. Pour the vegetable soup and bring to a boil. Cover with medium heat and cook for about 15 minutes or until all liquid is absorbed. Remove from heat and set aside with cover.
4. Heat the oil in a small skillet over medium heat. Put onion and boil for15 minutes till translucent. Stir the garlic and cook for another minute.
5. Heat the oven to 350 ° F.
6. Add quinoa, beans, corn, pepper, additional adobo sauce, chili powder, cumin, and salt to a large bowl. Mix well. Pour to full each pepper with 1/4 of the stuffing and put them in casserole to hold them snug. Bake for 15-20 minutes.

Cashew sauce

7. Add all ingredients to blender and mix until smooth. Turn this blended mixture into a saucepan. Cook over medium heat and stir until the sauce is slightly thicker. It takes about 5-10 minutes.

Assembly

8. Remove the stuffed peppers from the oven and pour all the cashew sauce.

DAY 5

BREAKFAST: CARROT CAKE TWO-BITE BALLS

Active Time: 20 minutes
Total Time: 20 minutes
Yield: 16 balls

Protein: 8 grams per serving (2 balls)

Carrot cake! I kid you not. Everything for a carrot cake is in here, all rolled up into perfect little balls. You can roll some in coconut and leave others plain. They are so pretty.

INGREDIENTS

- 1 cup old-fashioned oats
- ½ cup almond meal
- ½ cup pecans
- ⅓ cup plus 2 tablespoons of unsweetened shredded coconut, split
- 3 medium carrots, grated
- 15 dates, pitted
- 2 tablespoons unsweetened cocoa powder
- 2 tablespoons almond butter
- 1 teaspoon ground cinnamon
- ½ teaspoon ground nutmeg
- ½ teaspoon ground ginger

INSTRUCTIONS

1. Add the oats, almond meal, pecans, ⅓ cup coconut, carrots, dates, and cocoa powder to a food processor. Mix on high until well processed. You may need to sharpen the edge several times to confirm the dates aren't clumping. Add the almond butter,

cinnamon, nutmeg, and ginger. Mix again until well mixed. Scrape down again if needed.

2. Transfer to a flat surface and make sure all is blended well. Use your hands if necessary. Remove in pieces the dough and wrap into sixteen balls. Roll the balls in additional shredded coconut, if desired.

LUNCH: MIXED BAG CHOCOLATE WALNUT PROTEIN BARS

Active Time: 20 minutes
Cook time: 35 minutes
Total Time: 55 minutes
Yield: 8 YIELD

Protein: 9 grams per serving

The long slim bars will have you happily chewing your way to protein enrichment on your way out the door.

INGREDIENTS

- 3 tablespoons peanut butter
- 3 tablespoons maple syrup
- 1½ tablespoons coconut oil
- 1 tablespoon ground chia seeds
- 1¼ cups quick-cooking oats
- ½ cup walnuts
- ½ cup dairy-free chocolate chips
- ⅓ cup coconut sugar
- ¼ cup raw shelled hempseed
- 3 tablespoons protein powder
- ½ teaspoon ground cinnamon
- ¼ teaspoon salt

INSTRUCTIONS

1. Preheat the oven to 350°F.
2. Prepare an 8-inch square baking dish with parchment paper coming up on the sides on two opposite ends. Not over the top, just the sides. This makes for easier removal.
3. Add the peanut butter, maple syrup, and coconut oil to a small saucepan. Heat to melt the peanut butter and stir well. Take off heat and let cool a bit.
4. Mix the ground chia seeds and 3 tablespoons water in a small bowl and set aside.
5. Add the oats, walnuts, chocolate chips, sugar, hempseed, protein powder, cinnamon, and salt to a large bowl. Mix well. Add the chia mixture and peanut butter mixture to the bowl of dry ingredients and mix well.
6. put the mixture together in the bowl and press down with your fingers to make the mix firm and pressed into all corners.
7. Bake for 30 to 35 minutes. The bars will get harder as they cool, so don't overbake.
8. Let cool on a wire rack. To remove, grab hold of the extra parchment paper on the opposite ends of the dish and lift. Cut into bars that are about 2 inches wide and then in half at 4 inches long.

DINNER: PROTEIN POTLUCK SPECIAL

Active Time: 10 minutes

Cook time: 25 minutes

Total Time: 35 minutes

Yield: 8 YIELD

Protein: 36 grams per serving

Comfort food for the whole party! Whether for your family or made as a dish to go, this high-protein meal is the whole package.

INGREDIENTS

- 1 pound lentils
- 1 bay leaf
- 1 tablespoon extra virgin olive oil
- 1 cup finely chopped onion
- 1 green bell pepper, diced
- 2 carrots, finely chopped
- 3 Roma tomatoes, diced
- 1 teaspoon paprika
- 1 teaspoon ground cumin
- ½ teaspoon garlic powder
- ½ teaspoon onion powder
- 1 teaspoon coconut sugar
- ½ teaspoon salt

INSTRUCTIONS

1. Put the bay leaf and lentils in a big saucepan and cook according to package directions.
2. Apply heat to oil over medium-high heat in a very large skillet while cooking the lentils. Add the onions and bell pepper and sauté for 10 minutes. Add the remaining ingredients and sauté for 5 minutes. Add the lentils, stir, and cook for 5 minutes to heat through.

DAY 6

BREAKFAST: LEMON STRAWBERRY PROTEIN MUFFIN
Active time: 15 minutes

Cook Time: 25 minutes
Total time: 40 minutes
Yield: 6 YIELD

Protein: 10 grams per serving (1 muffin)

With big fat muffins for satiety and satisfaction, ensure the Strawberry is added for a contrasting fruity touch that we all covet many times.

INGREDIENTS:

- 2 tablespoons crushed chia seed or chia seed, split
- 5 tablespoons butter without dairy
- ½ cup coconut sugar
- ½ cup + 2 tablespoons dairy free milk
- 1 tablespoon lemon juice
- 1.5 cups whole wheat flour
- 1.5 teaspoons of baking powder
- 1/2 teaspoon baking soda
- 1/4 teaspoon salt
- ¼ cup raw cannabis with shell
- Half strawberry, chopped

INSTRUCTIONS:

1. Preheat oven to 375 ° F.
2. Grease the inside of a 6-cup muffin can and set aside.
3. Mix 1 tablespoon ground chia seed and 3 tablespoons water and save.
4. Using an electric mixer, mix the butter and sugar in a large bowl for about 3 minutes until lightly fluffy. Position the chia seed

mixture and stir again while adding milk and lemon juice. Mix well.
5. Add flour, baking powder, baking soda, salt, cannabis, and the remaining tablespoon of chia seeds to a medium bowl. mixture. Put the flour mixture to the saturated mixture and tap until just bonded. It becomes a sticky batter. Fold the strawberries.
6. Divide the batter into muffin cups. Fill at least three quarters, even if one cup is underfilled. Bake for 25 minutes, or until the nail tooth branch inserted in the center is clean.

Protein: 10 grams per serving (1 muffin)
Active time: 15 minutes
COOK TIME: 25 minutes
Total time: 40 minutes

LUNCH: PEANUT BUTTER SNACK SQUARES
Active Time: 10 minutes
Cook time: 20 minutes
Total Time: 30 minutes
Yield: 8 YIELD

Protein: 14 grams per serving (2 squares)

A double peanut whammy is served up in this recipe. All is sweetened with whipped coconut sugar and dates.

INGREDIENTS

- ½ cup coconut sugar
- 1 cup creamy peanut butter
- 1 teaspoon vanilla extract
- ¾ cup whole wheat flour
- ¼ cup garbanzo flour

- 1 teaspoon baking soda
- ½ teaspoon baking powder
- 1 cup old-fashioned oats
- ½ cup dairy-free milk
- ½ cup peanuts
- ½ cup dates, pitted and chopped small

INSTRUCTIONS

1. Preheat the oven to 350°F. Lightly grease an 8-inch square baking dish.
2. Mix the sugar and peanut butter over medium speed with a hand or stand mixer for 5 minutes. Mix the coffee in with it. Add the flours, baking soda, baking powder and mix at medium velocity. Pour in the oats and mix for a couple of seconds. This is going to be rigid. Add the milk and blend until just mixed on a medium.
3. Wrap in the peanuts and dates to make sure that everything is well set in.
4. You can use your hands to gently press the dough into the shaped platter. Bake for 20 minutes till golden brown is light.
5. Place to cool onto a wire rack. Cut into seventeen squares, and store in the fridge.

DINNER: SOUTHWEST VEGGIE-PACKED SALAD BOWL

Active Time: 20 minutes
Cook time: 25 minutes
Total Time: 45 minutes
Yield: 2 YIELD

Protein: 24 grams per serving

Vibrant colors fill this bowl with all the best vegetables associated with the Southwest. Add a small sweet potato and a spicy dressing and you're all set.

INGREDIENTS

Vegetables

- 1 small sweet potato, peeled and chopped in bite-size pieces
- 2 tablespoon extra virgin olive oil, divided
- ½ cup green lentils
- ½ cup diced red onion
- ½ cup diced bell pepper, orange and yellow
- ½ cup canned kidney beans, drained and rinsed
- 1 ear corn on the cob, kernels cut off of cob
- 1 teaspoon salt

Dressing

- ¼ cup extra virgin olive oil
- ¼ cup lime juice
- 2 tablespoons maple syrup
- ¼ to ½ teaspoon hot sauce
- ½ teaspoon salt

To Assemble

- 2 cups mixed lettuce
- ½ cup grape tomatoes, sliced in half

INSTRUCTIONS

Vegetables

1. Preheat the oven to 400°F.
2. Put the sweet potato on a baking sheet and sprinkle with 1 tablespoon oil and toss. Roast for about 25 minutes or until you can pierce the sweet potato easily with a fork
3. While the sweet potato is roasting, rinse the lentils. Add 1 cup

water and the lentils to a medium saucepan. Cover, bring to a boil, crack lid, and turn down the heat to medium. Cook about 20 minutes or until the lentils are tender.

4. Meanwhile, heat 1 tablespoon oil in a skillet applying an average heat. Put the onion and bell pepper together for 10minutes and sauté or until the onion is translucent. Add the kidney beans and corn and heat through. Stir in the lentils, sweet potato, salt, and set aside.

Dressing

5. Ensure all the ingredients for the dressing are mixed together and set aside afterwards.

Assembly

6. Divide the lettuce between two salad bowls, pulling the lettuce up higher on half of the bowl. Divide the lentil mixture between each bowl, filling up half the bowl. Lay a row of sliced grape tomatoes between the lettuce and vegetable mixture. Serve with the dressing.

DAY 7

BREAKFAST: HIGH PROTEIN CHOCOLATE BLENDER MUFFIN

Active time: 15 minutes
Cook time: 20 minutes
Total time: 35 minutes
Yield: 6 YIELD

Protein: 14 grams per serving (2 muffins)

These wet chocolate muffins are not guilty. Blend, pour and bake for an easy path to chocolate protein.

INGREDIENTS:

- 1 15 oz black beans, drain, rinse
- ½ cup of apple sauce
- 2 tablespoons
- ¼ cup milk without dairy
- 1 tablespoon lemon juice
- ½ cup maple syrup
- 2 teaspoons of vanilla essence
- 1 tablespoon flax seed
- ½ cup of unsweetened cocoa powder
- 1 teaspoon baking powder
- 1/2 teaspoon baking soda
- ½ cup of traditional oats
- ½Chop dairy free chocolate chips
- ¼ cup raw cannabis with shell

INSTRUCTIONS:

1. Preheat oven to 350 ° F.
2. Line up the paper liner in a 12 cup muffin can.
3. Put all ingredients except chocolate chips and hemp seeds into the blender. Blend until the mixture is as smooth as possible. Add the chocolate chips and hemp seeds and mix for 5 seconds or until dispersed.
4. Pour into muffin cups and fill at least three quarters. Bake for 20 minutes. After cooling for 5 minutes, move the paper cup to a wire rack to cool completely.
5. Store in refrigerator for up to 3 days or freeze for up to 6 months.

LUNCH: PUMP UP THE POWER ENERGY BALLS
Active Time: 20 minutes
Total Time: 20 minutes
Yield: 32 balls

Protein: 10 grams per serving (3 balls)

No-bake treats are so easy to make. Currants are readily available, and they seem to have been made to be combined with pepitas . . . and hempseed . . . and peanut butter . . .

INGREDIENTS

- 1 cup old-fashioned oats
- ¾ cup almond meal
- ⅓ cup wheat germ
- ¼ cup flaxseed meal
- ¼ cup pepitas
- 2 tablespoons raw shelled hempseed
- 1 teaspoon ground cinnamon
- ¼ teaspoon ground nutmeg
- ½ cup dried currants
- ½ cup peanut butter
- ⅓ cup maple syrup
- 1 teaspoon vanilla extract
- ¼ teaspoon salt

INSTRUCTIONS

1. Mix the oats, almond meal, wheat germ, flaxseed meal, pepitas, hempseed, cinnamon, nutmeg, and currants together in a medium bowl.
2. Add the peanut butter, maple syrup, vanilla, and salt to the bowl

of a stand mixer. Mix on medium speed until well combined. Pour the dry ingredients into the wet mixture. Mix on low until well combined.

3. Roll into thirty-two balls.

DINNER: PORTABELLA MUSHROOM GYRO

Active Time: 15 minutes

Cook time: 15 minutes

Total Time: 30 minutes

Yield: 2 YIELD

Protein: 16 grams per serving

Big fat marinated Portavera is a dream ingredient. Just wrap in flavored drops and spinach and add the best white sauce.

INGREDIENTS

Vegetables

- 2 large portabella mushroom caps
- 2 tablespoons vegan Worcestershire sauce
- 1 teaspoon ground cumin
- 1 teaspoon maple syrup
- ½ teaspoon dried oregano
- 1 tablespoon coconut oil
- ¼ cup diced red onion
- ½ red bell pepper, diced large
- Fresh White Sauce
- ½ cup vegan mayonnaise
- ¼ cup raw shelled hempseeds
- 1 tablespoon lemon juice
- ¼ teaspoon dried mint
- ¼ teaspoon dill weed

To Assemble

- 2 pita flatbreads
- 1 ounce baby spinach

INSTRUCTIONS

Vegetables

1. Remove the stem from the mushroom and remove the gills with a spoon. throw away. Cut the mushrooms thick.
2. Mix Worcestershire sauce, cumin, maple syrup and oregano in a medium bowl. Place the mushroom slices in the marinade and marinade for 10 minutes.
3. Heat the oil on a medium high heat in a large frying pan. Add the onions and peppers and fry for 10 minutes. Add the marinated mushroom slices and fry for an additional 5 minutes. Remove from heat and cool.

Fresh white sauce

4. Mix all the fresh white sauce ingredients in a small bowl and set aside.

Assembly

5. Place a layer of spinach leaves on each flatbread. Spoon a fresh white sauce in the middle. Place the mixture of mushrooms and peppers on top. Fold each flatbread and secure it with a decorative pick.

DAY 8

BREAKFAST: CHOCOLATE BANANA HEMP SMOOTHIE BOWL

Active time: 10 minutes

Total time: 10 minutes

Yield: 1 serving

Protein: 23 grams per serving

I'm just hiding a little spinach in a chocolate banana smoothie bowl. Make it for breakfast and you are heading for the running start of the day.

INGREDIENTS:

- Smoothie bowl
- 1 frozen banana, 4 slices for topping
- ½ cup almond milk or other dairy-free milk
- 1 tablespoon almond butter
- 1 tablespoon cocoa powder
- 1 tablespoon maple syrup
- 1 cup spinach
-

Topping

- 4 banana slices (from above)
- Strawberries and slices
- 2 tablespoons dairy-free chocolate chips
- 2 tablespoons of raw

INSTRUCTIONS:

1. Add smoothie bowl ingredients to blender and blend until smooth.
2. Pour into bowl and decorate with toppings.

LUNCH: SEITAN SLOPPY JOES

Active Time: 10 minutes

Cook time: 20 minutes

Total Time: 30 minutes

Yield: 6 YIELD

Protein: 26 grams per serving

A rich barbecue sauce and enriched seitan make for a much-loved sandwich. Hold it over a plate and have a big bite. Now *that's* good!

INGREDIENTS

- 2 cups seitan, crumbled (Slow Cooker Log for Thin Slices and Crumbles)
- 8 ounces tomato sauce
- ⅓ cup organic ketchup
- 1 tablespoon vegan Worcestershire sauce
- 2 tablespoons red wine vinegar
- 2 tablespoons coconut sugar
- 6 toasted whole wheat buns

INSTRUCTIONS:

1. Add all of the ingredients except the buns to a large skillet. In an average heat, boil and Cook for 15 minutes. Serve on the toasted buns.

DINNER: PEANUT BUTTER CHOCOLATE SEED BALLS

Active Time: 15 minutes
Refrigerator Time: 30 minutes
Cook time: 25 minutes
Total Time: 1 hour 10 minutes
Yield: 16 YIELD

Protein: 7 grams per serving (3 balls)

Here are some perfect little bites that only have five ingredients. The delicious result gives you a nice firm ball. Simple and fast!

INGREDIENTS

- 16 ounces dairy-free chocolate chips
- ½ cup creamy peanut butter
- ½ cup raw shelled hempseed
- ½ cup unsweetened shredded coconut
- 1 cup sunflower seed kernels, pulsed fine in a mini food processor, divided

INSTRUCTIONS

1. Melt the chocolate in a double boiler. Stir in the peanut butter and blend well. Take off of the the heat and mix in the hempseed, shredded coconut, and ½ cup sunflower seeds. Refrigerate until the dough is firm enough to use a small cookie scoop, about 30 minutes.
2. Bring the dough out of the fridge and scrape out forty-eight balls. You can roll them into smoother balls with the palms of your hands. While they are still warm from rolling, roll them in the remaining pulsed sunflower seeds.
3. These will keep in the fridge for about 3 weeks and in the freezer for about 6 months.

DAY 9

BREAKFAST: SOUTHWEST SCRAMBLE BREAKFAST BURRITO

Active time: 10 minutes

Cook time: 15 minutes

Total time: 25 minutes

Yield: 2 YIELD

Protein: 41 grams per serving

This recipe is a step beyond scrambled tofu. Add the vegetables and spices for a while and wrap it around the tortillas. The result is both filling and special.

INGREDIENTS:

- 1 tablespoon dairy-free butter
- ½ red pepper diced in a cup
- ½ red onion cup diced
- 8 oz firm tofu, drained and pressed
- ½ Cup steamed citrus potato rinks, crushed
- 1 tbsp taco seasoning
- 1/2 teaspoon salt
- 2 tablespoons flax seed meal
- 2 large tortillas with germinated grains

INSTRUCTIONS:

1. Dissolve butter in a large skillet over medium high heat. Add peppers and onions and fry for 10 minutes. Crush the tofu with the prepared seitan. Stir for another 5 minutes, add taco seasoning and salt. Sprinkle the flaxseed meal and mix well.
2. Spoon half of the mixture into each tortilla and roll into a burritos. Serve in half.

LUNCH: MULTI-LAYER AVOCADO TOAST

Active time: 15 minutes

Cook Time: 5 minutes

Total time: 20 minutes

Yield: 2 YIELD

Protein: 16 grams per serving

Avocado toast fills the breakfast brunch. Toasts topped with protein, fiber, and flavor make a simple breakfast sufficient for morning snacks.

INGREDIENTS:

- 1 tablespoon dairy-free butter
- 4 oz firm tofu, drained and pressed
- ¼ teaspoon black salt
- ¼ teaspoon onion powder
- Turmeric pinch
- 1 avocado
- Pinch of ground black pepper
- 1 teaspoon lime juice
- 2 slice sprouted grain bread

INSTRUCTIONS:

1. Add butter to a frying pan and heat over medium high heat. Crush the tofu in a frying pan. Sprinkle salt, onion powder and turmeric for about 4 minutes to make sure the tofu is broken into small pieces.
2. In a small bowl, mash the avocado with pepper and lime juice.
3. Toast the bread. Spread half of the prepared avocado on each part of the toast. Top with half of the prepared tofu on each piece of toast. Slice the toast diagonally in half.

DINNER: ULTIMATE VEGGIE WRAP WITH KALE PESTO

Active Time: 30 minutes

Soaking Time: 2 hours

Cook time: 10 minutes

Total Time: 2 hours 40 minutes

Yield: 2 YIELD

Protein: 24 grams per serving

Pretty in green on the inside and out. Tender broccoli and fresh veggie layers add to the flavorful kale pesto before you roll these up for your first bite.

INGREDIENTS

Kale Pesto

- ¼ cup of raw cashew nuts, soaked for at least 2 hours
- 1 cup kale, coarsely chopped with stem removed
- 1 clove garlic
- ½ teaspoon salt
- 2 tablespoons nutritional yeast
- 3 tablespoons extra virgin olive oil

Wrap

- ½ cup broccoli florets
- 2 spinach tortillas
- ¼ cup grated carrots
- ¼ cup diced red onion
- ½ yellow bell pepper, diced
- 6 ounces spinach
- 2 tablespoons raw shelled hempseed
- 2 tablespoons sunflower seed kernels

INSTRUCTIONS

Kale Pesto

1. Place the cashews, kale, garlic, and salt in a small food processor. Process for about 30 seconds, add the nutritional yeast and oil and process a few more seconds until well blended. Set aside.

Assembly

2. Add water to a medium-sized pan with a steamer and cook while

adding broccoli to it. Steam mixture in boiling water for ten minutes, Remove from the steamer and set aside.
3. Lay out the spinach tortillas. Divide the kale pesto between the two tortillas and spread evenly, leaving about 1 inch around all edges. Divide the remaining ingredients in half and lay out each half next to each other and down the length of each tortilla.
4. Start to roll up snugly, without tearing the tortilla. Cut each tortilla in half and serve.

DAY 10

BREAKFAST: GRANOLA WITH SEEDS, NUTS AND FRUITS
Active time: 10 minutes
Cook Time: 40 minutes
Total time: 50 minutes
Yield: 8 YIELD

Protein: 16 grams per serving

This recipe is stored in abundant quantities for about a month. Cereals stuffed with protein in the morning are a great way to start the day, especially if it's as easy as pouring into a bowl. With plant-based milk, you can add even more protein.

INGREDIENTS:

- 7 cups of traditional oats (use gluten free if needed)
- 1 cup shredded coconut
- 1 cup sunflower seed kernel
- 1 cup walnut
- 1 cup coconut sugar
- ¼Cup chia seed

- 1 cup coconut oil
- 1 cup raisin

INSTRUCTIONS:

1. Preheat oven to 300 ° F.
2. Mix all ingredients except raisins. Spread into a large baking pan.
3. Bake for 40 minutes. Remove from the oven and stir every 10 minutes. Return to the oven.
4. After 30 minutes, add the raisins and stir. Bake for another 10 minutes. Remove from oven and let cool.
5. Put in an airtight container. Hold for 4 weeks.

LUNCH: RICH CHOCOLATE ENERGY COOKIES

Active Time: 15 minutes
Cook time: 15 minutes
Total Time: 30 minutes
Yield: 12 YIELD

Protein: 6½ grams per serving (2 cookies)

These rich energy cookies are big and chewy, and a wonderful variety of ingredients goes into them. They won't stay in your cookie jar for long.

INGREDIENTS

- ½ cup dairy-free butter, softened
- 1 cup coconut sugar
- 1 tablespoon chia seeds or ground chia seeds
- 2 cups (12 ounces) dairy-free chocolate chips, divided
- 1 tablespoon instant coffee
- 1¼ cups whole wheat flour

- ½ teaspoon baking soda
- 1 teaspoon baking powder
- ½ teaspoon salt
- 2 tablespoons raw shelled hempseed
- 1 cup walnuts, chopped

INSTRUCTIONS

1. Preheat the oven to 350°F. Cut parchment paper on a baking sheet to match. put aside. 2. To pan, add butter and sugar a stand mixer. Cream on medium speed for 5 minutes or until light and fluffy.

3. Mix the chia seeds with 3 tablespoons water and set aside.

4. Melt ½ cup of the chocolate chips in a microwave or in a double boiler. Set aside to cool a bit.

5. Boil 2 tablespoons water and add instant coffee. Set aside to cool.

6. Add flour, baking soda, baking powder, and salt to a bowl. Mix well by hand.

7. Add the prepared chia seed mixture and melted chocolate to the bowl of the stand mixer. Mix well on medium speed. Add the flour mixture and keep mixing until just combined. Put away the bowl and wrap in the remaining chocolate chips, hempseed, and walnuts. Mix well.

8. Drop on the prepared cookie sheet by large, heaping tablespoons, 2 inches apart, and flatten slightly. Bake for 12 minutes.

9. Cool on a wire rack.

DINNER: PANAN SEITAN CURRY

Active time: 20 minutes

Cook Time: 45 m minutes
Total Time: 1 hour 5 minutes
Yield: 6 YIELD

Protein: 26 grams of protein per serving

Add all of the peanut sauce, red curry paste, and a small amount of hot sauce to make the key elements of this citrus and vegetable feast sweet and spicy.

INGREDIENTS:

- 1 cup red quinoa
- 1 sweet potato, peeled and cut into bite-sized pieces
- 1 tbsp extra virgin olive oil
- 1 red pepper diced
- ¼Chop finely chopped shallot
- 2 garlic cloves
- ¼Cup creamy peanut butter
- 2 tablespoons red curry paste
- 1 teaspoon of Sriracha
- 2 tsp turmeric
- 1 teaspoon of raw g
- 1 teaspoon cumin
- 14 oz can coconut cream
- 1 tablespoon lime juice
- 1/2 teaspoon salt
- 2 cup pressure cooker Thai nugget

INSTRUCTIONS:

1. Sift the quinoa and rinse well. Put the quinoa in a medium pot

and cover with 2 cups of water. Bring to a boil and then reduce heat to cover. Cook for about 15-20 minutes or until all the water is absorbed and the quinoa is soft. Set aside and covered.

2. Add water to a medium-sized pan with a steamer and bring to a boil. Add the sweet potato to the insert and steam in boiling water for 10 minutes.
3. Apply heat to oil in a big skillet over average heat. Add peppers and fry for 10 minutes. Add shallot and garlic and cook for 2 minutes. Add peanut butter, red curry paste, sriracha, turmeric, ginger and cumin. Cook for 5 minutes, stirring occasionally. Add 1 cup of water, coconut cream, lime juice and salt and mix. Add sweet potatoes and sycamore nuggets. Stir to medium heat. Reduce boiling and cover the fire with low heat. Cook for 10-15 minutes.
4. Serve with quinoa.

DAY 11

BREAKFAST: A TOUCH OF THE TROPICS RICE BOWL
Active Time: 15 minutes
Cook time: 10 minutes
Total Time: 25 minutes
Yield: 2 YIELD

Protein: 21 grams per serving
The repertoire requires rice. A great way to enjoy many kinds of fruits and vegetables, This rice introduces the taste of the tropics.

INGREDIENTS
Bowl

- 1 sweet potato, peeled and cut into bite-sized pieces
- 1 tbsp extra virgin olive oil
- 2 cups jasmine rice
- 1 pineapple, peel, core and chop to bite size
- ¼Cup cashew nut
- 4 tablespoons raw

Sweet and Sour Sauce

- 1 tablespoon cornstarch
- ½ cup chopped pineapple
- ¼ cup rice vinegar
- ⅓ cup light brown sugar
- 3 tablespoons ketchup
- 2 teaspoons soy sauce

INSTRUCTIONS

Sweet Potato

1. Preheat the oven to 425ºF.

2. Throw the oil over the sweet potato. Place them on a baking sheet and fry for 30 minutes.

3. Remove from the pan and let cool.

Nice sauce and sour 4. In a small bowl, mix cornstarch and a spoonful of water, Make a deposit.

5. Pour pineapple and 1/4 cup of water into the mixer. Blend as smoothly as possible until mixing is complete.

6. Put pineapple paste, rice vinegar, brown sugar, ketchup and soy sauce in a medium-sized pan. Bring to a boil over medium heat. Attach the cornstarch mixture and cook for about 1 minute until thick. Remove from heat and set aside

Assembley

7. Put rice in each bowl below. Removes clusters of bananas,

cashews, sweet potatoes, and hemp seeds, on a sweet and sour sauce.

LUNCH: SLOW COOKER POTATO TACOS
Active time: 15 minutes
Cook Time: 4 hours
Total time: 4 hours 15 minutes
Yield: 4 YIELD

Protein: 20 grams per serving (2 tacos)

Slow cookers don't make life so easy. The following is a list of rare **INGREDIENTS**s that exclude these tacos from the chart. There is no guessing what is included.

INGREDIENTS:

- 2 15 oz canned beans, drain, rinse
- 1 cup of fresh, frozen or canned corn
- 3 oz tipo pepper (approximately 2 peppers) in adobo sauce, chopped
- 6 oz tomato paste
- ¾Cup Thai sweet chili sauce
- 1 tablespoon sugar-free cocoa powder
- 1.5 tsp taco seasoning
- 8 white corn taco shells or tortillas or favorites
- Favorite toppings: spinach, lettuce, black olives, lime, avocado, peppers

INSTRUCTIONS:

1. Put everything except the taco shells and toppings into the clock

pot. Cook on low heat for 3-4 hours and on high heat for 1.5-2 hours.

2. Spread a considerable amount of filling, whether hard or soft, on the taco shell. Add your favorite toppings.

DINNER: BROCCOLI TOFU QUICHE

Active time: 30 minutes

Immersion time: 1 hour

Cook Time: 50 minutes

Total time: 2 hours 20 minutes

Yield: 6 YIELD

Protein: 21 grams of protein per serving

Elegance and protein are wrapped in this beautiful quiche. A special dinner full of vegetables and completely reheated. This quiche can be baked in a spring-foamed bread or pie dish.

INGREDIENTS

- ¼ cup of raw cashew nuts, soaked for 1 hour
- ½ cup of water
- Nutritional yeast 1 tablespoon
- 2 tablespoons tapioca flour
- 1 tablespoon red miso
- 1/2 teaspoon cider vinegar
- 1/4 teaspoon salt
- ¼ teaspoon garlic powder

Quiche

- 1 tbsp extra virgin olive oil
- 1 cup spinach
- ½ red onion cup diced
- 1 cup of diced red peppers (about 1 pepper)

- 8 oz cremini mushrooms, sliced
- 1½ cup broccoli, the inner stem is cut into cubes, and the florets are cut into bites
- 3 pieces of garlic, finely chopped
- 1 cup of canned black beans, drain, rinse
- 16oz solid tofu, drained and pressed
- ¼ cup milk without dairy
- ¼ teaspoon turmeric
- 2 tsp oregano
- 1 tsp salt
- ¼ teaspoon ground black hu pepper
- One package vegan pie crust including two crusts

INSTRUCTIONS

1. Add all ingredients to the blender. Mix until smooth.

2. Pour into a small pot and cook on medium to high heat. It gets thicker and becomes slightly elastic within 5 minutes. If you think it is too thick to combine with the quiche ingredients, you can add one drop of water at a time. Set aside.

Quiche

3. Preheat oven to 350 ° F.

4. Heat the oil over medium heat in a large skillet. Add the spinach and cook until wilted. Remove from bread and set aside. Add the onions, peppers, mushrooms and broccoli to the pan and fry for about 10-15 minutes until the onions are translucent. Put garlic and boil for some minutes then add black beans and stir. Pour into a large mixing bowl.

5. Divide the tofu into a blender and add milk, cashew, turmeric, oregano, salt and pepper. Blend as smoothly as possible. Add the mixture to the stir-fried vegetables and mix well.

6. Pour into one pie crust. Cover with a second pie crust and crimp the ends. If using a spring foam pan, make a rounded edge on the

bottom skin and place the top skin on top of the **INGREDIENTS**. Bake the quiche for 30 minutes.

DAY 12

BREAKFAST: A COLLECTION OF THAI SEITAN AND VEGETABLES

Active time: 15 minutes

Cook time: 30 minutes

Total time: 45 minutes

Yield: 6 YIELD

Protein: 19 grams per serving

This is a fold mix of all the best vegetables and the most popular vegetables. Tasty citrus is added and all the spices make this jumbled pop flavorful.

INGREDIENTS:

- 2 carrots, sliced
- 1 small cauliflower cut into small flowers
- 1 small broccoli
- 1 tbsp extra virgin olive oil
- 1 diced white onion
- One red pepper, Julian
- 8 oz mushrooms, sliced
- 1 cup pressure cooker Thai nugget
- ¼ teaspoon time
- ¼ teaspoon basil
- 1/2 teaspoon salt
- ¼ teaspoon ground black hu pepper

INSTRUCTIONS:

1. Add water to a medium-sized pan with a steamer insert and bring to a boil. Add carrot and cauliflower and steam with boiling water for 5 minutes.
2. Add broccoli on cauliflower and steam for another 10 minutes. Pick all the vegetables and make sure they can be easily stabbed with a fork. Do not overheat. Al dente is best.
3. Apply heat to oil in a big frying pan. Add the onions and peppers and fry for 10 minutes. Add the mushrooms to the pan and cook for another 10 minutes. Add seitan nuggets and all herbs and spices. Stir and heat for about 2 minutes. Add the cauliflower mixture, stir well and cook for another 5 minutes.

LUNCH: CHOPPED CHICKPEA SALAD VEGGIE BOWL

Active Time: 20 minutes

Cook time: 15 minutes

Total Time: 35 minutes

Yield: 2 YIELD

Protein: 17 grams per serving

This is a delicious dish that incorporates chickpea salad. There's lots of roughage, too, that just begs for the simple balsamic dressing.

INGREDIENTS

Quinoa

- ½ cup dry quinoa
- 1 cup vegetable broth
- Pinch of salt
- Chickpea Salad

- 1 15-ounce can chickpeas, drained and rinsed
- ¼ cup vegan mayonnaise
- 1 tablespoon nutritional yeast
- 1 tablespoon cider vinegar
- ½ teaspoon ground mustard
- 2 scallions, finely sliced
- 1 teaspoon salt
- Pinch of cayenne pepper

Dressing

- ½ cup extra virgin olive oil
- ¼ cup balsamic vinegar

To Assemble

- 3 cups chopped romaine lettuce
- ½ cup diced purple cabbage
- ½ cup diced orange bell pepper

INSTRUCTIONS

Quinoa

1. Sift the quinoa and rinse well. Mix the quinoa, soup and salt in a small pot. Bring to a boil, cover and boil down. Cook for 15 minutes or until the soup is absorbed. Remove from heat and set for 5 minutes with cover attached. Remove the lid and put it in a fluffy small bowl to cool.

Chickpea salad

2. Put all the ingredients of the chickpea salad into the food processor. Pulse 4-5 times. Chickpeas should be thick. Remove the blade and stir so that the mixture is well mixed.

Dressing

3. Mix the oil and vinegar together in a small bowl and set aside.

Assembly

4. Divide the lettuce between two bowls. Lay the vegetables in decorative rows: cabbage, quinoa, bell pepper, and chickpea salad, leaving an edge of romaine lettuce. Serve with the dressing.

DINNER: ARTICHOKE FLATBREAD WITH CRUSHED CITRUS

Active time: 20 minutes

Immersion time: 1 hour

Cook Time: 10 minutes

Total time: 1 hour 30 minutes

Yield: 2 YIELD

Protein: 39 grams per serving

You have to make this! Flatbread topped with these simple ingredients will be a great deal of pleasure and protein.

INGREDIENTS

- Cashew
- Soak the cup of raw cashew nuts for 1 hour to overnight and drain
- ½ cup of water
- Nutritional yeast 1 tablespoon
- 1 tablespoon tapioca starch or tapioca flour
- 1/2 teaspoon of garlic
- 1/2 teaspoon onion
- 1 tablespoon lemon juice

To assemble

- 2/ 8 inch flatbread
- ¼ cup spinach, cut into strips
- Steamed Seitan Smoky Nugget in a cup
- 14 oz artichoke water

- 1 tomato, chopped
- ¼Canned sliced black olives in a cup
- Raw shelled cannabis for topping

INSTRUCTIONS:

Cashew

1. Add all ingredients to blender and mix until smooth. Turn this blended mixture into a saucepan. Cook over medium heat and stir until the sauce is slightly thicker. It takes 5-10 minutes. Let cool and take heat.

Assembly

2. Spread a 1/2 cup layer of cashew on each flatbread. Sprinkle half of spinach on each flatbread. Separate citrus, artichoke, tomato and olives and sprinkle evenly on each flatbread.
3. Sprinkle on top with hemp seeds.

DAY 13

BREAKFAST: BREADED AND BAKED CAULIFLOWER TEMPETACOS

Active time: 15 minutes
Marinating time: 1 hour
Cook time: 30 minutes
Total time: 1 hour 45 minutes
Yield: 4 YIELD

Protein: 30 grams per serving (2 tacos)

Now is the time for all the good cooks to bake the crumbly cauliflower. The flavor has so many layers that the two are easy to use.

INGREDIENTS:

- 8 oz original tempe
- 3 tablespoons hot sauce (such as Frank)
- ¼ In addition to a cup, 2 tablespoons sugar-free dairy-free milk, split
- 1 small head cauliflower
- 1 cup whole wheat flour
- 2 tablespoons taco seasoning
- Panco bread crumb cup
- Nutritional yeast 2 tablespoons
- 1 tablespoon coconut oil
- Lomin lettuce 2 cups
- 8 taco shell
- 2 tomatoes, chopped
- Lime wedge (optional)
- Salsa (optional)

INSTRUCTIONS:

1. Preheat oven to 350 ° F.
2. Cut the tempe into ¼-inch strips across the width and tear them into approximately ½-inch pieces.
3. Mix 1 tablespoon of hot sauce and 2 glasses of milk in a small bowl. Add tempe and toss. Marinate for one hour.
4. Meanwhile, cut the small flowers into bite-sized pieces to prepare cauliflower.
5. Mix 2 tablespoons hot sauce and 1/4 cup milk in a large bowl. Add cauliflower and toss.
6. Add flour, taco seasoning, panco and nutritive yeast to a large bowl and mix well.
7. Remove the cauliflower from the wet mixture, add it to the flour mixture and coat all florets. Place on a baking sheet, bake for 20-30

minutes, spin after 15 minutes. When done, you can easily drill holes with a fork.

8. While baking the cauliflower, heat the oil in a small skillet over medium high heat and add tempe. Cook for about 2 minutes, occasionally turn over and bake until the pieces turn golden. Move from heat to paper towel.

9. Put the lettuce on the bottom of the shell, put the tempe, cauliflower and tomato with a spoon to assemble the taco. If needed, add lime wedges and salsa.

DINNER: KALE THROW'S THREE-LAYER TACO

Active time: 25 minutes

Total time: 25 minutes

Yield: 3 YIELD

Protein: 30 grams per serving (2 tacos)

With these overflowing tacos, you'll want a taco night every night. The tofu is marinated with pinto beans and the spicy, sweet slaw acts as a topping.

INGREDIENTS:

filling

- 1 tbsp taco seasoning
- 3 tablespoons
- 8 oz solid tofu, drainer, press, cut into ½ inch chunks
- 1 15 oz can focus, drain and rinse beans
- ¼ Cup fine onions
- Two diced roman tomatoes
- 1/2 teaspoon salt

- Pinch of ground black pepper
- 1 teaspoon chopped parsley

Kale Throw

- 1 cup coarsely chopped kale with stalks removed
- 1 tablespoon lemon juice
- 1 cup thin sliced purple cabbage
- 1 cup thinly sliced green cabbage
- ¼ cup carrot
- 2 tablespoons dairy free mayonnaise
- 1 tablespoon lime juice
- 1 tsp maple syrup
- 1 chopped pepper of finely chopped advo sauce

To assemble

- 6 taco shell

INSTRUCTIONS:

filling

1. Mix taco seasoning and puddle in a small bowl. Set aside.
2. Add the tofu to the pool mix and toss. Marinate bean mixture and throw during work.
3. Put beans, onions, tomatoes, salt, hu pepper and parsley in a small bowl. Throw and melt.

Kale Throw

4. Add kale to a medium bowl and add lemon juice. Massage the kale by hand to soften it. Add cabbage, carrots, mayonnaise, lime juice, maple syrup and chili advo sauce. Mix well.

assembly

5. Assemble the tacos by layering the husks with a bean mixture, tofu and finally throw.

LUNCH: RICH MUSHROOM GRAVY AND POLENTA
Active time: 20 minutes
Cook Time: 45 minutes
Total time: 1 hour 5 minutes
Yield: 4 YIELD

Protein: 22 grams per serving

Polenta is strange and easy to make. Enjoy a meal with plenty of mushroom gravy.

INGREDIENTS:
Polenta

- ¼ cup coconut oil
- 1 tablespoon chopped shallot
- 3 pieces of garlic
- 1 teaspoon dried basil
- Dry white wine cup such as Chardonnay
- 3 cups vegetable soup
- chopped Roman tomato
- 1/2 teaspoon salt
- 1 cup cornmeal
- Mushroom gravy
- 2 tablespoons extra virgin olive oil
- 1 pound button mushroom, slice
- 1 tablespoon chopped shallot
- 1 piece of garlic finely chopped
- 3 tablespoons flour
- 2 cups vegetable soup
- 1/2 teaspoon salt
- ¼ teaspoon ground black hu pepper

- 1 cup pressure cooker tender patties, crumbled

INSTRUCTIONS:

Polenta

1. Grease a 9 inch square pan.
2. Heat the coconut oil in a large pot over medium high heat. Add the shallots and cook for 3-5 minutes or until tender. Add the garlic and basil and cook for another minute. Stir the wine and bring to a boil. Reduce heat and cook for 5 minutes. Add soup, tomatoes and salt. Bring to a boil, reduce heat and add cornmeal. Cook and stir for 15-20 minutes or until the polenta has thickened and pulled off the side of the pan.
3. Pour into prepared pan and spread evenly in all four corners. Set aside for cooling to room temperature. This takes about 20-30 minutes.

Mushroom gravy

4. Make mushroom gravy while polenta is cold. Heat the olive oil in a frying pan. Add mushrooms and fry for 10-15 minutes. Add shallot and fry for 3-5 minutes. Add the garlic and flour and cook for another minute. Add vegetable soup, salt and pepper. Bring to a boil and then over medium heat, cook for about 5 minutes or until slightly thicker. Add the crushed putty, cook for another 5 minutes and heat.
5. Slice the polenta into squares, and add 1-2 slices to a plate with mushroom gravy on top.

DAY 14

BREAKFAST: TORTA DE SEITAN AND VEGGIES

Active Time: 45 minutes

Cook time: 25 minutes

Total Time: 1 hour 10 minutes
Yield: 4 YIELD

Protein: 31 grams per serving

So difficult to let fork out of skillet when this spicy mix is being prepared. Fill up those rolls and have a great lunch.

INGREDIENTS

- 1 tablespoon coconut oil
- ½ cup diced red onion
- 1 green bell pepper, diced
- 2 cloves garlic, minced
- ½ teaspoon dried oregano
- ½ teaspoon ground cumin
- 4 Steamed Seitan Chipotle Links
- 1 15 oz black beans, drain, rinse
- 2 sub rolls
- 1 cup salsa
- Romaine lettuce, sliced and chopped

INSTRUCTIONS

1Heat up the oil over medium to high temperature in a large skillet and Stir in the onion and bell pepper and sauté for 10-15 minutes or until golden brown

Stir in the garlic, oregano, cumin and roast for 1 minute. Tear the seiten into chunks and drop into the skillet. Add the black beans. Stir and cook over medium heat for 5 minutes or until seitan is heated through.

2. Half cut the roll and scrap some of the bread center. Spread a layer of salsa on the bread and sprinkle on some chopped romaine

lettuce. Fill up with black bean and seitan mixture.

LUNCH: LAYERED OAT AND CHOCOLATE BARS
Active Time: 20 minutes
Cook time: 5 minutes
Refrigerator time: 1 hour
Total Time: 1 hour 25 minutes
Yield: 16 squares

Protein: 7 grams per serving (1 square)

You wouldn't think that no-bake bars could look like this and hold together like this, but they do. They're more like a candy bar than anything else, except they're loaded with protein.

INGREDIENTS

- 1 cup dairy-free butter
- ½ cup coconut sugar
- 1 teaspoon vanilla extract
- 3 cups quick-cooking oats
- ¼ cup raw shelled hempseed
- 2 tablespoons protein powder
- 1 cup dairy-free chocolate chips
- ½ cup peanut butter

INSTRUCTIONS

1. Position an 8 "square baking platter with baking parchment paper and come up about 3 inches on opposite sides. This will act as a handle to remove the squares from the dish.
2. In a medium saucepan, melt the butter over medium-high heat. Add the sugar and vanilla. Mix the in oats and cook for 2 minutes. Add the hempseed and protein powder and mix well. Pass half the mixture to the ready one dish and press firmly and evenly into all

edges and corners.
3. Place the chocolate and peanut butter in a small saucepan. Heat over low heat until chocolate is melted and all is well combined. Pour over the bottom layer in the prepared dish and smooth evenly all over the top. Crumble on top of what is left in the oat mixture as evenly as possible and lightly press into the chocolate.
4. Refrigerate for at least 1 hour.
5. Grab the "handles" of the parchment paper and lift out of the dish. Place on a cutting sheet and slice into sixteen squares.

DINNER: AMAZING LENTIL ENERGY BALLS
Active Time: 15 minutes
Refrigerator Time: 30 minutes
Cook time: 25 minutes
Total Time: 1 hour 10 minutes
Yield: 9 YIELD

Protein: 12 grams per serving (4 balls)

What?! Lentil balls as a sweet protein snack, you say? Yes, it's possible. They're sweetened just right—try them once and you'll be craving them forever. No kidding!

INGREDIENTS

- ½ cup lentils
- ½ cup dairy-free chocolate chips
- 2 cups quick-cooking oats
- ¼ cup sunflower seed kernels
- ¼ cup raw shelled hempseed
- ¼ cup unsweetened shredded coconut
- ½ cup almond butter
- ½ cup maple syrup

INSTRUCTIONS

1. Rinse lentils, and drain them. In a medium-large saucepan, place 1 cup of water and the lentils. After high heat bring to a boil. Turn down to medium height when the water comes to boil, and cook for 25 minutes or until the lentils are soft. We should consume all of the vapor. Set aside to freshen up.
2. In a large bowl incorporate the chocolate chips, peas, sunflower seeds, hempseeds, and coconut. Add in refrigerated lentils. Add the butter for almond and the maple syrup. Blend well. Shape into thirty-six balls, and put them with a lid in a glass container.
3. Chill for about 30 minutes. Store for up to 5 days in the refrigerator, or freeze for up to 6 months.

DAY 15

BREAKFAST: BLACK BEAN PATTIES WITH CARROTS AND CORN

Active Time: 15 minutes

Cook time: 20 minutes

Total Time: 35 minutes

Yield: 6 YIELD

Protein: 22 grams per serving

Treat yourself to one of the most popular sandwiches out there. An added bonus is that this version has little bits of carrots and corn.

INGREDIENTS

- 1½ cups breadcrumbs, fresh
- 2 tablespoons of chia seed or ground chia seed
- 2 tablespoons coconut oil, divided

- 1 cup diced yellow onion
- ½ cup finely diced carrot
- 1 ear of corn, kernels cut from the cob, or 1 8-ounce can corn, drained
- ½ teaspoon dried oregano
- 2 teaspoons chili powder
- ¼ teaspoon ground cumin
- 1 teaspoon salt
- 2 cloves garlic, finely diced
- 1 28-ounce can black beans, drained and rinsed
- ¼ cup sunflower seed kernels
- 2 tablespoons raw shelled hempseed
- 6 whole wheat buns
- Condiments and toppings of your choice

INSTRUCTIONS

1. Make your breadcrumbs using any leftover bread that you have. I used whole wheat but you could use sourdough and whatever else you prefer. Place bread in a food processor and process until the bread is a finely ground texture. Set aside. If you have any leftover breadcrumbs, they can be frozen for 6 months.
2. Mix the chia seeds with 6 tablespoons water and set aside.
3. Apply heat to a tsp oil in a big skillet, add the onion and carrot, and sauté about 10 minutes. Add the corn and cook another 3 minutes. Add the spices and garlic to the onion and cook another minute.
4. Pat the black beans dry. When mashing and adding the remaining ingredients, you need to make sure they are not wet. In a large bowl, add black beans and a mash behind a potato masher or fork. Pulse them in a food processor instead, but not too fine. Stir in the chia seed mixture. Mix in the onion mixture,

breadcrumbs, sunflower seed kernels, and hempseed.
5. Make into six patties. After freeze the patties before frying
6. Fry the patties in 1 tablespoon medium-hot oil until browned on each side.
7. Serve on the whole wheat buns with your favorite toppings.

LUNCH: CRAZY QUINOA PROTEIN MUFFIN
Active time: 15 minutes
Cook Time: 35 minutes
Total time: 50 minutes
Yield: 6 YIELD

Protein: 7 grams per serving (1 muffin)

These cute muffins are crispy on the outside and cake-like on the inside. Sweeten with raisins and maple syrup to seduce you anytime.

INGREDIENTS:

- ½ Cup quinoa
- 2 tablespoons chia seed or chia seed
- ¼ cup almond flour
- 3 tablespoons of vanilla protein powder
- 1/2 teaspoon salt
- ½ Cup date, small increments
- 2 tablespoons coconut oil
- 3 tablespoons maple syrup
- 1 teaspoon of vanilla essence
- ¼ cup of unsweetened shredded coconut
- ½ cup raisins

INSTRUCTIONS:

1. Put quinoa in an medium small pot with a lid after rinsing. Cover with a cup of water and boil over medium high heat. Cover and lower. Cook for 20 minutes and remove from heat. Remove the lid and let it cool.
2. Preheat oven to 450 ° F. Line up six muffin cups and paper liners.
3. Mix the ground chia seeds with ¼ cup and 2 tablespoons of water and save.
4. Add almond flour, protein powder and salt to a small bowl. Mix well. Add the date and mix on the coat. Set aside.
5. Put the coconut oil in a medium bowl. If not liquid, heat in a microwave for 10-20 seconds or until dissolved. Remove from microwave and add maple syrup. Stir well. When cool, add the chia seed mixture, vanilla extract, coconut and almond flour mixture, cooked quinoa and raisins. Mix well.
6. Divide the batter between the six muffin cups and bake for 12-15 minutes until the nail p branch inserted in the center is clean.

DINNER: SPROUTED GRAIN SPICY SEITAN SANDWICH

Active Time: 5 minutes

Cook time: 10 minutes

Total Time: 15 minutes

Yield: 6 YIELD

Protein: 15 grams per serving

This super simple sandwich stars tender patties from an Instant Pot or pressure cooker. Premake the seitan and keep in the fridge or freezer for a super fast lunch.

INGREDIENTS

1 tablespoon coconut oil

- 6 Pressure Cooker Tender Patties
- 6 sprouted grain English muffins, sliced open
- Condiments of your choice, such as dairy-free chipotle mayo and horseradish mustard
- 1 avocado, sliced
- 6 slices red onion

INSTRUCTIONS

1. Steam the oil in a big skillet over an average-high heat and fry the patties until just golden on each side.
2. While the patties are in the skillet, toast the English muffins. Layer the toast with mayo, mustard, avocado, patty, and onion.

DAY 16

BREAKFAST: BROCCOLI SPINACH STUFFED BAGUETTE
Active Time: 45 minutes
Soaking Time: 1 hour
Cook time: 25 minutes
Total Time: 2 hours 10 minutes
Yield: 2 YIELD

Protein: 31 grams per serving

A soft gooey cashew with broccoli and spinach is added. Fill up a baguette hollowed out, and it's a feast.

INGREDIENTS

Vegetables

- 2 cups of broccoli flower
- 1 tablespoon of extra virgin olive oil
- 2 cloves of garlic, finely diced
- 5 ounces of baby spinach, sliced, with long stems cut away and discarded
- Cashew , 1/2 cup of raw cashew, soaked 1 hour and drained
- 1 cup of water
- 11/2 teaspoons of nutritional yeast
- 4 tablespoons of tapioca
- 1/2 teaspoon of salt
- 1/2 teaspoon of garlic powder

To prepare 1 baguette 1 ounce of grapefruit

INSTRUCTIONS

1. Add water with a steamer applied to a medium saucepan, and bring to a boil. Add the broccoli to the pipe, and steam 10 minutes over boiling water. Remove, and set aside from the steamer.
2. Steam up the oil over medium to high heat in a large skillet. Use a skillet that comes with a top. Add the garlic and boil for 1 minute. Stir in the spinach, toss, and simmer 1 minute. Cover for 2 minutes, and let sit.
3. Remove the spinach and broccoli to a large bowl.

Cashew food

4. Apply all the ingredients of cashew to a blender and combine until completely smooth.
5. Pour into a small saucepan and add medium - high pressure. Keep cooking and stirring until its thickening process is complete and becomes a gooey, salty sauce. It takes between 5 and 10 minutes.
6. Add the broccoli mixture to the pot. Shake good.
7. Cut off the baguette top and use a spoon to scoop out some of

the bread from the bottom. Make sure you leave a bread edge inside the shell to help hold the filling.

8. Spoon the broccoli mixture into the baguette core. Using sliced grape tomatoes to cover and scatter with hempseed. Half-cut. You may cut into slices as well, and serve as an appetizer.

LUNCH: PEPITA AND ALMOND SQUARES

Active Time: 20 minutes

Cook time: 15 minutes

Refrigerator Time: 30 minutes

Total Time: 1 hour 5 minutes

Yield: 16 squares

Protein: 12 grams per serving (2 squares)

Almonds and pepitas are two of the highest protein–packed seeds and nuts around. Combine them with even more powerhouse ingredients and you've got a very healthy little package.

INGREDIENTS

- 1 cup almonds, coarsely chopped
- 1 cup old-fashioned oats
- ⅔ cup pepitas
- ⅔ cup dried cranberries
- ½ cup unsweetened shredded coconut
- ¼ cup raw shelled hempseed
- ⅓ cup peanut butter
- ⅔ cup brown rice syrup
- ¼ cup maple syrup
- 2 teaspoons vanilla extract

INSTRUCTIONS

1. cover the square baking bowl with parchment paper and come up about 3 inches on opposite sides. This will act as a handle to remove the squares from the dish.
2. In a large mixing bowl, add the almonds, oats, pepitas, cranberries, coconut, and hempseed. Mix well. Stir in the peanut butter and try to get it evenly combined. You can use your fingers when most of it is worked in.
3. Add the brown rice syrup, maple syrup, and vanilla to a small saucepan. Bring to a boil and continue boiling until it reaches the hard ball stage, 260°F, on a candy thermometer. When this temperature is reached, quickly pour over the almond mixture and stir well. It will start to harden up quickly. Pour into the prepared dish and press down firmly into the dish and as evenly as possible. Refrigerate for at least 30 minutes.
4. Grab the "handles" of the parchment paper and lift out of the dish. Place on a cutting sheet and slice into sixteen squares.

DINNER: SEITAN AND SUN-DRIED TOMATO PESTO VEGGIE SANDWICH

Active Time: 20 minutes

Cook time: 20 minutes

Total Time: 40 minutes

Yield: 2 YIELD

Protein: 28 grams per serving

Thick slices of special seitan and tender cauliflower make the best sandwich when combined with pesto and spinach. After all is encased in a folded flatbread, it simply begs for a bite.

INGREDIENTS

Cauliflower

- 1 tablespoon extra virgin olive oil
- ½ cup cauliflower florets
- Pinch of salt
- Sun-Dried Tomato Pesto
- ¼ cup baby spinach, packed
- Fill two tablespoons of sun-dried tomatoes with oil and drain. (Save the oil)
- 1 tablespoon pine nuts
- 1 clove garlic
- 2 teaspoons nutritional yeast
- Pinch of garlic powder
- ¼ teaspoon salt
- 1 tablespoon oil or reserved oil from the sun-dried tomatoes

To Assemble

- 2 slices flatbread
- 1 ounce baby spinach
- ¾ cup Slow Cooker Maple Breakfast Links, sliced
- 2 slices red onion

INSTRUCTIONS

Cauliflower

1. Preheat the oven to 425°F.
2. Sprinkle the oil on a baking sheet. Lay the cauliflower on the oil and sprinkle with salt. Toss with your hands to get the oil dispersed onto the cauliflower. Bake for 20 minutes or until the cauliflower can be pierced easily with a fork, Remove and set side.

Sun-Dried Tomato Pesto

3. Ensure all pesto ingredients are together in a small food

processor, starting with the spinach. Process until well blended.
Assembly

4. Lay out the flatbreads. Spread half the pesto on each flatbread. Divide the spinach, seitan, cauliflower, and onion between the flatbread slices. Fold each flatbread and secure it with a decorative pick.

DAY 17

BREAKFAST: FRESH VEGGIE SEITAN PITA POCKET
Active Time: 15 minutes
Cook time: 5 minutes
Total Time: 20 minutes
Yield: 2 YIELD

Protein: 35 grams per serving

Fresh vegetables and tender seitan fill up these pita pockets for a memorable lunch.

INGREDIENTS

- 1 tablespoon extra virgin olive oil
- 1 cup Steamed Seitan Smoky Nuggets, sliced thick
- ½ cup broccoli florets, chopped small
- ½ cup diced red bell pepper
- ½ cup diced cucumber
- 1 carrot, grated
- 4 ounces artichoke hearts in water, drained
- 2 pita pockets
- ¼ cup dairy-free mayonnaise

- 1 ounce baby spinach

INSTRUCTIONS

1. Steam the oil in a big saucepan over moderate to high steam. Add the seitan, broccoli, and bell pepper and cook over medium heat for 3 minutes. Add the cucumber, carrot, and artichoke hearts. Stir and cook for 1 minute. Take off the heat.
2. Cut the pita pockets in half and spread half the mayonnaise into both halves of each pocket. Include baby spinach leafs and then spoon a quarter of the seitan mixture into each of the four pocket halves.

LUNCH: CHERRY CHOCOLATE HEMP BALLS

Active Time: 20 minutes
Total Time: 20 minutes
Yield: 24 balls

Protein: 10 grams per serving (2 balls)

Take a gander down this list of ingredients. Every nut, grain, fruit, and seed included here just makes me happy. They blend so well together, and they freeze perfectly, too.

INGREDIENTS

- 1 cup old-fashioned oats
- ½ cup unsweetened shredded coconut
- ½ cup dried cherries, chopped
- ½ cup pistachios, chopped
- ⅓ cup dairy-free chocolate chips
- ⅓ cup peanut butter
- ¼ cup maple syrup

- ¼ cup raw shelled hempseed

INSTRUCTIONS

1. Add all of the ingredients to a large bowl. Mix well with a sturdy wooden spoon. Roll into 24 balls.
2. keep in the refrigerator which could be as long as 5 days or freeze for up to 6 months.

DINNER: SPROUT SANDWICH WITH TOFU RICOTTA

Active Time: 30 minutes

Total Time: 30 minutes

Yield: 2 YIELD

Protein: 26 grams per serving

A nice thick layer of homemade tofu ricotta and sun-dried tomato pesto make a terrific sandwich. Add even more veggies for a unique and delicious lunch.

INGREDIENTS

- Sun-Dried Tomato Pesto
- ¼ cup baby spinach, packed
- Fill two tablespoons of sun-dried tomatoes in oil and drain. (Save oil)
- 1 tablespoon pine nuts
- 1 clove garlic
- 2 teaspoons nutritional yeast
- Pinch of garlic powder
- ¼ teaspoon salt
- 1 tablespoon oil or reserved oil from the sun-dried

tomatoes

- Tofu Ricotta
- 7 ounces extra-firm tofu, drained, pressed and crumbled
- 1 tablespoon extra virgin olive oil
- 1 teaspoon cider vinegar
- 1 teaspoon lemon juice
- ½ teaspoon garlic powder
- ½ teaspoon onion powder

To Assemble

- 4 slices sprouted grain bread
- 1 cup alfalfa sprouts
- 1 Roma tomato, sliced
- 2 slices red onion
- Pinch of garlic powder

INSTRUCTIONS

Sun-Dried Tomato Pesto

1. In a food processor add all the ingredients starting with the spinach. Process until well blended.

Tofu Ricotta

2. Place all the ricotta ingredients in a small food processor. Process until well blended.

Assembly

3. Spread a thick layer of the tofu ricotta on two bread slices. Apply pesto on the other two slices of bread.Divide the sprouts, tomato, and onion and place on the ricotta. Top with the pesto slice. Slice each sandwich into fourths in triangle shapes.

DAY 18

BREAKFAST: VANILLA ALMOND DATE BALLS

Active Time: 20 minutes

Total Time: 20 minutes
Yield: 20 balls

Protein: 8 grams per serving (2 balls)

Vanilla is such a great flavor, and it seems to make something a treat without going over the top. Almond flour and protein powder is added for an extra oomph of protein.

INGREDIENTS

- 1½ cups almond flour
- 16 dates, pitted
- 4 tablespoons sunflower seed kernels
- 4 tablespoons vanilla protein powder
- 2 tablespoons flaxseed meal
- 1 teaspoon vanilla extract
- Pinch of salt
- 2 tablespoons sunflower seed kernels, ground fine in a small food processor

INSTRUCTIONS

1. Place all the ingredients except the ground sunflower seeds in a food processor. 2. Process on high until all is combined well and forms a ball. Transfer into a large bowl and form twenty balls. This dough works well by squeezing each one a few times to form a ball. Roll in ground sunflower seeds.

LUNCH: PRESSURE COOKER THAI NUGGETS
Active Time: 10 minutes
Cook time: 5 minutes
Rest Time: 1 hour

Total Time: 1 hour 15 minutes
Yield: 4 YIELD

Small unformed nuggets with delectable flavors come from your pressure cooker with this recipe. They have an Asian flair and can be added to just about any recipe.

Protein: 30 grams per serving (½ cup)

INGREDIENTS:

- ¾ cup plus 3 tablespoons vital wheat gluten
- ¼ cup chickpea flour
- ½ teaspoon ground ginger
- ½ teaspoon salt
- ¼ teaspoon garlic powder
- ¼ teaspoon paprika
- ¾ cup vegetable broth
- 2 teaspoons tamari, divided
- 4 teaspoons red curry paste, divided
- 1½ cups vegetable broth, divided

INSTRUCTIONS

1. Add the gluten, flour, ginger, salt, garlic powder, and paprika to a large bowl.
2. Mix ¾ cup vegetable broth, 1 teaspoon tamari, and 2 teaspoons red curry paste in a small bowl. Throw all the mixture that is wet into the mixtures that are dry.
3. Mix and then knead for about 2 to 3 minutes or until elastic. It's a very wet dough but you will see it is still elastic. It should be mildly stretchy and pull back but still pliable. Pinch off pieces of dough into very small balls, about 1 to 1½ inches in diameter. They

will fatten up when cooking.

4. Place in an electric pressure cooker.

5. Add 1½ cups vegetable broth, 1½ cups water, and 2 teaspoons red curry paste to a bowl and stir well. Pour over the nuggets in the pressure cooker. Close the lid and make sure you spin the top knob to lock. Click Manual at pot end. Press button to 4 (that means 4 minutes). The pressure cooker will give a click and the pressure will begin to build. Building pressure, and cooking, will take about 15 minutes. Leaving the nuggets to fall in the pot. They are going to cook more as the pressure of course releases. Don't wind.

6. Go ahead and vent after about an hour. It may have already completely cooled, but vent to ensure that the pressure has been released and then open the lid.

7. Take the nuggets off the liquid and set aside to cool. You will quickly eat them, add them to a recipe or keep in the fridge overnight. They are great the next day. You can also freeze them.

DINNER: PESTO AND CRISPY TOFU FLATBREAD SANDWICH

Active Time: 15 minutes

Soaking Time: 1 hour

Cook time: 40 minutes

Total Time: 1 hour 55 minutes

Yield: 2 YIELD

Protein: 33 grams per serving

Multiple textures and flavors galore make this sandwich a prime target for your regular recipe rotation.

INGREDIENTS

Tofu

- 2 ounces extra-firm tofu, drained, pressed, and cut into 1-inch cubes
- ¼ cup vegetable broth
- 1 tablespoon tamari
- 1 teaspoon onion powder
- ¼ teaspoon salt
- ¼ cup cornstarch

Pesto

- ¼ cup raw cashews, soaked for 1 hour
- 1 cup basil, packed
- 1 clove garlic
- ½ teaspoon salt
- 2 tablespoons nutritional yeast
- 3 tablespoons extra virgin olive oil
- To Assemble
- 1 tablespoon coconut oil
- ¼ cup diced onion
- 6 mushrooms, sliced
- ¼ cup hummus
- 2 slices flatbread
- ½ cup sunflower sprouts

INSTRUCTIONS

Tofu

1. Mix together the vegetable broth, tamari, onion powder, and salt in a small bowl. Add the tofu and let marinate at least 1 hour.
2. Preheat the oven to 350°F.
3. Place the cornstarch in a medium bowl.
4. Remove the tofu from the marinade and place it on cornstarch. Throw it and set it on the baking sheet. Bake for 30-40 minutes.

Turn around for 12 minutes till it becomes golden swelling.
Pesto
5. Place the cashews, basil, garlic, and salt in a small food processor. Process for about 30 seconds. Add the nutritional yeast and olive oil and process a few more seconds until well blended.
Assembly
6. Heat the coconut oil in a skillet over medium-high heat. Add the onions and mushrooms and sauté for about 10 to 15 minutes or until onion is translucent. Remove from the heat.
7. Spread half of the hummus on each flatbread. Spread half of the pesto on each flatbread. Sprinkle half of the tofu, sunflower sprouts, mushrooms, and onion down the center of each flatbread. Fold each flatbread and secure it with a decorative pick.

DAY 19

BREAKFAST: TROPICAL LEMON PROTEIN BITES
Active Time: 20 minutes
Total Time: 20 minutes
Yield: 24 balls

Protein: 8 grams per serving (2 balls)

You have to have a lemon treat in your bag of tricks. Easy to make, these balls don't fall apart or make any kind of a mess.

INGREDIENTS

- 1¾ cups cashews
- ¼ cup coconut flour

- ¼ cup unsweetened shredded coconut
- 3 tablespoons raw shelled hempseed
- 3 tablespoons maple syrup
- 3 tablespoons fresh lemon juice

INSTRUCTIONS

1. Place the cashews in a food processor and process until very fine. Add the rest of the ingredients and process until well blended. Dump the mixture into a large bowl.
2. Take a clump of the dough and squeeze it into a ball. Keep squeezing and working it a few times until a ball is formed and solid.

LUNCH: CHOCOLATE CAKE MUNCH COOKIES

Active Time: 10 minutes
Refrigerator Time: 1 hour
Cook time: 10 minutes
Total Time: 1 hour 20 minutes
Yield: 12 YIELD

Protein: 7 grams per serving (2 cookies)

Big, fat, and very chocolaty cookies are on the menu for today. Cake-like on the inside, they'll satisfy your cookie cravings any day.

INGREDIENTS

- ½ cup dairy-free butter, softened
- 1 cup coconut sugar
- 1 tablespoon chia seeds or ground chia seeds
- ¾ cup soy milk

- 1 teaspoon vanilla
- 2 cups whole wheat flour
- ¼ cup protein powder
- 1 teaspoon baking powder
- ½ teaspoon baking soda
- ½ teaspoon salt
- ½ cup cocoa powder
- 1 cup walnuts, chopped

INSTRUCTIONS

1. Add butter and sugar to the bowl of a stand mixer. Mix on medium speed for 5 minutes.
2. Meanwhile, mix the chia seeds with 3 tablespoons water.
3. Add the chia mixture, milk, and vanilla to the butter and mix well at medium speed.
4. Add the flour, protein powder, baking powder, baking soda, salt, and cocoa to a medium bowl. Mix well.
5. Turn mixer on medium and slowly add the dry mixture. Add the walnuts and mix at low speed until combined. Place the mixture in the refrigerator from one hour to overnight.
6. About 15 minutes before you're ready to bake the cookies, preheat the oven to 400°F. Cut parchment paper on a baking sheet to match. put aside

7. Drop heaping tablespoons onto prepared cookie sheet, 2 inches apart. Roll into balls and then flatten by about half with the bottom of a measuring cup or some other strong **INGREDIENTS**. They bake up thick. Bake for 8 minutes.
8. Cool on a wire rack.

DINNER: MIXED BEANS CHILI
Active Time: 10 minutes
Soaking Time: 8 hours
Cook time: 1 hour 30 minutes
Total Time: 9 hours 40 minutes
Yield: 6 YIELD

Protein: 20 grams per serving

How about some vegan chili that is comforting and full-flavored at the same time? It's made from scratch to warm you, your family, and your home.

INGREDIENTS

- 1 pound beans, mixed varieties (you can buy premixed or mix your own)
- 1 tablespoon extra virgin olive oil
- ½ cup diced onion
- 4 cloves garlic, finely chopped
- 4 cups vegetable broth, more if needed
- 1 28-ounce can crushed fire-roasted tomatoes
- 1 8-ounce can tomato sauce
- 1 6-ounce can tomato paste
- 2 tablespoons vegan Worcestershire sauce
- 2 tablespoons chili powder
- 2 teaspoons ground cumin
- 1½ teaspoons dried oregano
- ¼ teaspoon ground cloves
- ½ teaspoon cayenne pepper
- 1 teaspoon salt

INSTRUCTIONS

Before night

1. Rinse beans and place in large stock pot. Cover with about 3 inches of water. The beans swell. Soak overnight.

Next morning

2. Discharge the beans and return to the stock pot.
3. Heat the oil on a medium high heat in a large frying pan. Add the onions and saute until translucent (approximately 10-15 minutes). Add the garlic and fry for another minute. Add this mixture to the stockpot beans. Add the vegetable soup, crushed tomatoes, tomato sauce, tomato paste and Worcester sauce. Beans should be covered with a few inches of liquid. You can add broth or water as needed. Stir well. Add the remaining ingredients and mix again. Cover and bring to a boil.
4. Remove the lid, reduce the heat and cook over very low heat. Very low so the liquid hardly moves. Do not replace the lid. Remove the lid for more flavor. If the liquid is cooked to the point where the beans do not sink, add some soup or water. (If you add more liquid, re-cover, bring the heat to a boil, lower immediately and remove the cover.) Make sure the heat is not too high. Cook for 1 hour and check the beans. You will want to make them soft. If you have not done so, cook it longer. There is no need to cook for over an hour and a half.

DAY 20

BREAKFAST: PROTEIN POWER PISTACHIO BITES

Active Time: 15 minutes

Total Time: 15 minutes

Yield: 18 balls

Protein: 6 grams per serving (2 balls)

Who doesn't like pistachios? You can have these bites at a moment's notice, for yourself or friends. They're easy to pack along, too.

INGREDIENTS

- ½ cup old-fashioned oats
- ½ cup almond butter
- ¼ cup maple syrup
- ⅓ cup oat bran
- ⅓ cup flaxseed meal
- ⅓ cup pistachios, ground
- 1 tablespoon raw shelled hempseed

INSTRUCTIONS

1. Put all the ingredients in a big bowl and mix well.
2. Roll into eighteen balls.

LUNCH: ORANGE CRANBERRY POWER COOKIES

Active Time: 15 minutes
Cook time: 10 minutes
Total Time: 25 minutes
Yield: 12 YIELD

Protein: 6 grams per serving (2 cookies)

Mild fruit flavors blend perfectly in this sweet cookie dough. You'll feel like celebrating when you bite into one of these lightly crispy cookies.

INGREDIENTS

- 1 cup dairy-free butter, softened
- 1 cup coconut sugar
- ⅓ cup orange juice
- 2 teaspoons organic vanilla extract
- 1½ cups whole wheat flour
- 2 tablespoons protein powder
- 1 teaspoon baking powder
- ¼ teaspoon baking soda
- 1 cup old-fashioned oats
- 1 cup dairy-free chocolate chips
- 1 cup walnuts, chopped
- 1 cup dried cranberries

INSTRUCTIONS

1. Preheat the oven to 375°F.
2. Beat the butter and sugar together in the bowl of a stand mixer. Add the orange juice and vanilla extract. Mix well.
3. Add flour, protein powder, baking powder, and baking soda to a medium bowl. Mix and add to the wet mixture. Mix on medium speed until well blended. Add the oats, chocolate chips, walnuts, and cranberries. Mix on low.
4. Drop heaping tablespoons about 2 inches apart on an ungreased baking sheet. These are big cookies. They spread out to 3 to 4 inches in diameter. Bake for 10 to 11 minutes.
5. Cool a minute and then transfer to a wire rack to cool completely.

DINNER: ROASTED ROOT VEGETABLE SALAD BOWL
Active Time: 15 minutes

Cook time: 35 minutes
Total Time: 50 minutes
Yield: 2 YIELD

Protein: 24 grams per serving

Here's the perfect bowl to get a good helping of vegetables. Simply roast a few root vegetables and then chop a few more veggies to create this healthy power bowl. It's perfect with a nutty sweet tahini sauce.

INGREDIENTS

Roasted Vegetables

- 1 peeled sweet potato
- 1 parsnip, peeled and sliced into ¼-inch rounds
- 2 carrots, peeled and sliced into ½-inch rounds
- 2 tablespoons extra virgin olive oil
- ½ teaspoon salt
- Tahini Dressing
- ¼ cup tahini
- 1 tablespoon maple syrup
- 1 tablespoon lemon juice
- 1 clove garlic
- ¼ teaspoon salt
- Pinch of ground black pepper
- 3 tablespoons water

To Assemble

- ¼ cup diced red onion
- ½ cup chopped red cabbage
- 9 ounces baby spinach
- ¼ cup raw shelled hempseed

- 1 tablespoon chia seeds, black or white

INSTRUCTIONS

Roasted Vegetables

1. Preheat the oven to 375°F.
2. Place the sweet potatoes, parsnips, and carrots on a baking sheet, keeping them separated. Drizzle the oil over the top and lightly toss, still keeping the vegetables separated. Sprinkle with salt. Bake till they can be pierced with a fork or for 35 minutes. Set aside.

Tahini Dressing

3. Add all the dressing ingredients to a blender and blend until smooth.

Assembly

4. Prepare the salad bowls by placing half the spinach in the bottom of each bowl. Arrange all the remaining vegetables and hempseed in a circle around the edge of the bowl. Pour half of the dressing in the center of the vegetable round. Sprinkle with the chia seeds.

DAY 21

BREAKFAST: CHOCOLATE TRAIL MIX BARS

Active Time: 20 minutes

Refrigerator Time: 30 minutes

Total Time: 50 minutes

Yield: 8 bars

Protein: 16 grams per serving (1 bar)

These big and sturdy bars are great for the trail or even for just sitting in the backyard. Melted chocolate is included, so they are nice and chocolaty, too.

INGREDIENTS

- ¾ cup old-fashioned oats
- ½ cup bran flakes cereal
- ½ cup mixed nuts, chopped
- ¼ cup dried cherries
- ¼ cup dried cranberries
- ¼ cup raw shelled hempseed
- 3 tablespoons peanut butter
- ¼ cup maple syrup
- ½ cup dairy-free chocolate chips, melted

INSTRUCTIONS

1. Position an 8 "square baking platter with baking parchment paper and come up about 3 inches on opposite sides. This will act as a handle to remove the bars from the dish.
2. Add the oats, cereal, nuts, cherries, cranberries, and hempseed to a large bowl and mix well.
3. Mix the peanut butter and syrup together and pour into the large bowl. Mix well. Add the melted chocolate and mix again.
4. Press firmly into the prepared dish and into all corners. Let set in the refrigerator for 30 minutes.
5. Grab the "handles" of the parchment paper and lift out of the dish. Place on a cutting board and slice down the center. Turn and make three even cuts, which will give you eight long bars.

LUNCH: CHOCOLATE SUNFLOWER PROTEIN COOKIES

Active Time: 15 minutes
Cook time: 10 minutes
Total Time: 25 minutes

Yield: 12 YIELD

Protein: 7 grams per serving (2 cookies)

Sunflower seeds and give these softly crunchy chocolate chip cookies a pleasant texture. Bake a few hundred for your belly and cookie jar.

INGREDIENTS

- 1 cup dairy-free butter
- ¾ cup plus 2 tablespoons coconut sugar
- 2 tablespoons ground chia seeds
- 2¼ cups whole wheat pastry flour
- ¼ cup protein powder
- 1 teaspoon baking soda
- ½ teaspoon baking powder
- ¼ teaspoon salt
- 1 teaspoon vanilla extract
- 1 cup dairy-free chocolate chips
- ¼ cup sunflower seed kernels

INSTRUCTIONS

1. Preheat to 375 ° F on burner. Cut parchment paper on a baking sheet to match. Deposit back.
2. Add the butter and sugar to the stand mixer bowl and blend for 5 minutes at medium-low speed.
3. Meanwhile, mix and set aside ground chia seeds with 6 spoonfuls of water.
4. In a medium bowl, add the flour, protein powder, baking soda, baking powder, and salt.
5. Attach the combination of vanilla and chia to the butter blend. Mix well until blended. A little at a time, mix in the flour mixture.

Mix the chocolate chips and the sunflower seeds at low speed.
6. Shape into round balls, and set about 2 inches apart on the prepared baking sheet. Flat to approx. 1/2 inch high. Bake for 8 to 9 minutes.
7. Cool on a wire rack.

DINNER: SMOKY TEMPEH BUDDHA BOWL
Active Time: 15 minutes
Cook time: 35 minutes
Total Time: 50 minutes
Yield: 2 YIELD

Protein: 15 grams per serving

A warm and colorful lunch is something worth your time. The ingredients in this bowl act as complements to each other, with the added bonus of protein.

INGREDIENTS
Bowl

- 1 small sweet potato, chopped into bite-size pieces
- 1 tablespoon extra virgin olive oil
- ½ teaspoon salt
- ¼ cup dry quinoa
- ½ cup vegetable broth
- 4 ounces faux bacon-flavored tempeh

Almond Curry Sauce

- 3 tablespoons almond butter
- 3 tablespoons dairy-free milk
- 1½ tablespoons tamari

- 1 tablespoon rice vinegar
- 1 tablespoon red curry paste

To Assemble

- 2½ cups baby spinach
- ½ cup chopped red bell pepper
- ½ cup chopped purple cabbage

INSTRUCTIONS

Bowl

1. Preheat the oven to 375°F.

2. Put the potatoes on the baking sheet. Put oil on the edge

3. Meanwhile, quinoa is cooking. Place the quinoa and rinse well with a sieve. Mix the quinoa and soup in a small pot. Bring to a boil, cover, and boil until simmered. Cook for 10-15 minutes or until the soup is absorbed. Remove from heat and set in cover for 5 minutes.

4. Cut the tempeh into 1/4 slices and then into cubes.

Almond curry

5. In a small bowl, mix all ingredients until smooth and well mixed.6. Fill each salad bowl with the spinach. Make a decorative rim with the spinach tips if so desired. Divide the quinoa and vegetables between the two bowls and lay in a circle: peppers, quinoa, cabbage, sweet potatoes, and lastly, tempeh. Drizzle the dressing in a circle over all.

DAY 22

BREAKFAST: APPLE BROCCOLI CRUNCH BOWL

Active Time: 20 minutes

Total Time: 20 minutes

Yield: 6 YIELD

Protein: 9 grams per serving

Here's a bowl that's filled with everyone's favorite vegetables and fruits. Mix all the ingredients inside a bowl then pour on the slightly sweet and tangy dressing. Toss and eat!

INGREDIENTS

Bowl

- 2 medium heads broccoli (about 4 cups when chopped)
- 3 sliced apples
- ¼ cup diced red onion
- ½ cup raisins
- ½ cup sunflower seed kernels
- ¼ cup raw shelled hempseed

Dressing

- ¼ cup cider vinegar
- ½ cup extra virgin olive oil
- 2 cloves garlic, minced
- 1 tablespoon maple syrup (you can use up to 2 tablespoons)
- ½ teaspoon salt
- ¼ teaspoon ground black pepper

INSTRUCTIONS

Bowl

1. Cut the florets from the broccoli stalks and set the stalks aside. Cut the florets into very small pieces. Place in a large bowl.
2. remove after slicing the hard external part of the skin away from the broccoli stalks to get down to the tender inside. Discard the

outer skin. Cut the inside stems into matchsticks. (Or you can use a mandolin or food processor that has an attachment that will cut the stems into long strips—not grated. The aim is to have very tiny points of raw broccoli stems that retain their form Remove the florets then remove to the large mixing bowl. Stir in the apples, onions, raisins, sunflower seeds, and hempseed.

Dressing

3. Mix and stir all dressing ingredients in a medium bowl. Introduce the salad dressing, and toss. Chill to fully prepare for serving.

LUNCH: DOUBLE-DECKER RED QUINOA SANDWICH

Active Time: 20 minutes

Cook time: 35 minutes

Total Time: 55 minutes

Yield: 3 YIELD

Protein: 24 grams per serving

A little preparation and a food processor takes you a long way to this satisfying sandwich. Red quinoa has the same nutty taste and nutrition of its pearly cousin, and it's just darn pretty.

INGREDIENTS

- ½ cup red quinoa
- 1 cup vegetable broth
- 4 large portabella mushroom caps
- 2 tablespoons coconut oil, divided
- ¼ cup finely chopped onion
- ½ cup raw pecans
- 2 green spring onions, chopped
- 2 teaspoons rice wine vinegar

- 1 teaspoon garlic powder
- 2 tablespoons nutritional yeast
- 2 tablespoons raw shelled hempseed
- ¼ cup flour
- 3 whole wheat burger buns

Toppings and condiments: lettuce, tomatoes, red onion, mustard, dairy-free spicy mayo.

INSTRUCTIONS

1. Sew the quinoa, then rinse properly. Mix the quinoa in a small pot and the soup. Bring to a boil and cover, then steam. Cook for 10-15 minutes, or until it consumes the broth, Remove from heat and put on cover for 5 minutes.
2. Drop gills and discard mushrooms. Chop a stem on the mushroom.
3. In a large frying pan, melt a spoonful of oil. Remove the mushrooms and onion, and fry for 10 minutes. Add the pecans and sauté for 5 more minutes. Remove from the heat and let cool.
4. Add the mushroom mixture, green onion, and vinegar to a food processor. Process until very fine. It will not be smooth.
5. move to a big bowl and mix quinoa, garlic powder, nutritional yeast, hempseed, and flour. Mix until well blended. Form into six patties the size of the burger buns.
6. Heat remaining oil in a large skillet and fry one patty at a time so that you can flip it easily. Fry until golden brown on each side.
7. Assemble the double deckers: Lay down the bottom of the bun, add mustard, lettuce, patty, red onion, lettuce, dairy-free spicy mayo, patty, dairy-free spicy mayo, tomatoes, and top of bun.

DINNER: VEGGIE STUFFED CALZONE
Active Time: 30 minutes
Rising Time: 90 minutes
Cook time: 25 minutes
Total Time: 2 hours 25 minutes
Yield: 2 YIELD

Protein: 21 grams per serving

This homemade calzone dough is stuffed with prepared veggies and a little of this and a little of that. Slide it in the oven to bake for a great lunch that you deserve.

INGREDIENTS

Dough

- 1 packet dry active yeast
- 1 tablespoon extra virgin olive oil
- ¾ teaspoon salt
- ¾ cup whole wheat pastry flour
- 1 cup unbleached all-purpose flour

Filling

- 2 cups broccoli florets
- 1 tablespoon extra virgin olive oil
- 1 red bell pepper, diced
- 1 cup cremini mushrooms
- ½ cup diced red onion
- 4 ounces artichoke hearts in water, drained
- 2 tablespoons chopped walnuts
- ½ teaspoon dried rosemary
- ¼ teaspoon salt
- ¼ teaspoon ground black pepper

- ½ cup vegan mayonnaise or spread of your choice
- 2 tablespoons dairy-free milk
- 2 tablespoons cornmeal

INSTRUCTIONS

Dough

1. Apply oil to the inside of a large bowl and set aside. This is because the dough rises.
2. Put a cup of warm water (100-110 ° F) into another large, heated bowl (you can warm the bowl with a microwave). Stir the yeast and leave for 10 minutes. Put water, oil and salt in a cup and mix. Stir until flour is added and mixed. Not smooth.
3. Move to a counter scrubbed with flour and knead for about 4 minutes until smooth. To avoid sticking, add a little more flour. A little sticky is OK. Become a ball. Place the dough ball in a large oiled bowl and turn the dough until all surfaces are greased. Failure to do this will result in a dry crust on the outside of the ball. Cover the bowl and let it sit (from the draft) for 40-60 minutes until the dough doubles in size.
4. Divide the dough in half. Half the dough is formed into two balls and placed on a floured counter. Cover with a towel again and raise for another 20-30 minutes.
5. On a lightly powdered surface, flatten and extrude the dough with your fingers, or use a rolling pin to form two circles of the same size (about 10 inches each). One is up and the other is down. Cover again with towels and rest for 10-15 minutes.

Filling

6. Add water to the medium-sized pan with the steamer, and bring to a boil. Put the broccoli and heat in boiling water for 10 minutes. Remove from the steamer and set aside.
7. Heat the oil over medium high heat in a large frying pan. Add red

peppers, mushrooms and onions and fry for 10 minutes. Add artichoke heart, walnuts, rosemary, salt and pepper and fry for another 5 minutes. Stir the broccoli and set aside.

Assembly

8. Preheat the oven to 425°F.
9. Uncover the calzone dough. Spread the mayonnaise on one dough round. Next spread the broccoli mixture, leaving about ½ to 1 inch of the edge not covered. Carefully lift the plain dough round and place on the broccoli-covered round. Press and fold the edges over. Cut a few slits in the top of the dough. Brush lightly with milk.
10. Spread the cornmeal on a baking sheet. Carefully lift the calzone onto the baking sheet. Bake for 15 to 18 minutes.
11. Cut the calzone as you would a pizza and serve.

DAY 23

BREAKFAST: NO-BAKE CEREAL DATE BARS

Active Time: 20 minutes
Cook time: 15 minutes
Refrigerator Time: 30 minutes
Total Time: 1 hour 5 minutes
Yield: 16 bars

Protein: 9 grams per serving (2 bars)

Layers of crunchy goodness are filled with so many wonderful sweet flavors. Not too sweet, though—these bars have just the right contrast and balance.

INGREDIENTS

- 2 cups granola cereal

- 2 tablespoons flaxseed meal
- 2 tablespoons protein powder
- ½ cup peanuts, chopped
- ½ cup dates, chopped small
- ½ cup almond butter
- ½ cup brown rice syrup
- ¼ cup maple syrup

INSTRUCTIONS

1. Cover square baking bowl with parchment paper and come up about 3 inches on opposite sides. This will act as a handle to remove the bars from the pan.
2. Combine the cereal, flaxseed meal, protein powder, peanuts, and dates in a large bowl.
3. In a small saucepan, add the almond butter and both syrups. Bring to a boil and cook to the hard ball stage, 260°F, on a candy thermometer. Quickly stir into the cereal mixture and then spread into the prepared dish. It will cool quickly, so you can use your fingertips to press down into the dish as evenly as possible. Refrigerate for at least 30 minutes.
4. Grab the "handles" of the parchment paper and lift out of the dish. Put it on a cutting board and slice into 16 squares.

LUNCH: PRESSURE COOKER TENDER PATTIES

Active Time: 10 minutes
Cook time: 5 minutes
Rest Time: 1 hour
Total Time: 1 hour 15 minutes
Yield: 2 cups

Protein: 30 grams per serving (½ cup)

These patties are ready in no time with an electric pressure cooker and are super simple to make. There seems to be an infinite number of recipe possibilities for these little disks.

INGREDIENTS

- ¾ cup vital wheat gluten
- ¼ cup chickpea flour
- 2 tablespoons nutritional yeast
- ½ teaspoon dried basil
- ½ teaspoon salt
- ½ teaspoon poultry seasoning
- ¼ teaspoon garlic powder
- ¼ teaspoon onion powder
- ¼ teaspoon paprika
- 2¼ cups vegetable broth, divided
- 1 teaspoon extra virgin olive oil
- ½ teaspoon tamari
- 2 tablespoons tomato sauce

INSTRUCTIONS

1. Add the gluten, flour, nutritional yeast, basil, salt, poultry seasoning, garlic and onion powders, and paprika to a large bowl.
2. Mix ¾ cup vegetable broth, oil, and tamari in a small bowl. Put together the wet mixture and the dry ingredients
3. Mix and then knead for about 2 to 3 minutes or until elastic. Ensure it is stretchy and pull back but still pliable. Divide the dough into eight pieces. Use your fingers to squeeze and work around into a patty measuring about 3 to 4 inches in diameter.
4. Place in an electric pressure cooker.
5. Add 1½ cups water, 1½ cups vegetable broth, and the tomato

sauce to a small bowl, stir, and then pour over the seitan cutlets in the pressure cooker. Close the lid and make sure to change the top knob to lock. Click Manual at pot end. Press button to 4 (meaning 4 minutes) The pressure cooker will make a click in a few seconds and start building up steam. Building pressure, and cooking, will take about 15 minutes. Leave the cutlets to set in the pot. They are going to cook more as the pressure of course releases. Don't wind.

6. Go ahead and complain after about an hour. It may have already completely cooled, but it vented to ensure that all the pressure was released and then opened the lid.

7. Extract from the liquid the cutlets and set aside for cooling. You can eat them immediately, add to a recycle, or keep in the fridge overnight. They are great the next day and keep well in the freezer.

DINNER: MINI PEPPER WITH STUFFED TEMPE CHICKPEAS

Active time: 20 minutes

Total time: 20 minutes

Yield: 6 YIELD

Protein: 9 grams per serving (2 peppers)

Colorful mini peppers wrap these protein-laden appetizers in small packages. Chickpeas and tempeh are just the beginning of a flavorful mix.

INGREDIENTS:

- 12 oz multicolor sweet mini pepper
- 2 oz canned chickpeas, drain, rinse
- ¾Cup tempe, chopped
- ½ cup dairy free mayonnaise
- ¼Cup cider vinegar

- 1 teaspoon mustard
- 3 sliced green onions
- 1 tsp salt
- ¼ teaspoon cayenne pepper

INSTRUCTIONS:

1. Cut off the end of the pepper stem. Slice vertically. Remove any species inside. Set aside.
2. Put all remaining ingredients into the food processor. Pulse 4-5 times. Chickpeas should be thick. Remove the blade and stir so that the mixture is well mixed.
3. Pack half the chickpea mixture in half. Serve on a plate.

DAY 24

BREAKFAST: STEAMED SEITAN SMOKY NUGGETS
Active Time: 10 minutes
Cook time: 40 minutes
Total Time: 50 minutes
Yield: 4 YIELD

Protein: 30 grams per serving (½ cup)

These smoky, savory bites make for a flavorful addition to an endless number of recipes. Robust in flavor, this small-batch recipe is also great when used as a sandwich filler. This is a densely textured seitan.

INGREDIENTS

- ¾ cup vital wheat gluten

- ¼ cup plus 2 tablespoons chickpea flour
- 2 teaspoons garlic powder
- 2 teaspoons onion powder
- ½ cup vegetable broth
- 2 tablespoons tomato sauce
- 1 tablespoon tamari
- 1 teaspoon liquid smoke
- ½ teaspoon coconut oil

INSTRUCTIONS

1. Add the gluten, flour, and garlic and onion powders to a large bowl.
2. Add the broth, tomato sauce, tamari, liquid smoke, and oil to a small bowl and mix well. Pour the liquid into the dry ingredients and mix. Knead for 2 minutes until elastic. You will see it pull back into a rounder shape as you knead. This is a firm dough and will not double in size while cooking.
3. Add 5 cups water to a saucepan. Bring to a boil. Position the steamer bowl inside the pan and turn down the heat to simmer.
4. Use a pastry cutter to slice off irregular pieces. You can squeeze them into a ball, as best you can, or leave chunky. You can also steam as one log and cut into chunks after steaming and cooling.
5. Steam for 40 minutes.
6. Remove the seitan to cool and store in the refrigerator for up to 5 days

LUNCH: STEAMED SEITAN CHIPOTLE LINKS

Active Time: 15 minutes

Cook time: 40 minutes

Total Time: 55 minutes

Yield: 1 cup or 4 links

Protein: 30 grams per serving (½ cup)

These spicy hot links can be fried and served as a link, or they can be sliced or crumbled. Regardless, they push so many recipes over the top. This is a small-batch recipe, so you can double the ingredients if you're looking for a larger quantity.

INGREDIENTS

- ⅓ cup plus 2 tablespoons vital wheat gluten
- 2 tablespoons chickpea flour
- 1 teaspoon garlic powder
- 1 teaspoon onion powder
- 1 teaspoon taco seasoning
- 2 tablespoons tomato sauce
- 1 teaspoon chipotle hot sauce

INSTRUCTIONS

1. Add the gluten, flour, garlic and onion powders, and taco seasoning to a large bowl.
2. Mix ¼ cup water, the tomato sauce, and hot sauce in a small bowl and mix well. Pour the liquid mixture into the dry ingredients and mix. Knead for 2 minutes until elastic. You will see it pull back into a rounder shape as you knead. This is a firm dough and will not double in size as cooking.
3. Cut into four equal pieces and roll each one into a log shape.
4. Add 5 cups water to a saucepan. Bring to a boil. Position the steamer bowl inside the pan and turn down the heat. Add seitan links to the steamer basket and cover. Steam for 40 minutes
5. Remove the seitan to cool and store in the refrigerator for up to 5 days

DINNER: FRIED HOISIN TOFU WITH PEANUT SAUCE–TOUCHED UDON

Active Time: 20 minutes

Marinating Time: 30 minutes

Cook time: 15 minutes

Total Time: 1 hour 5 minutes

Yield: 2 YIELD

Protein: 33 grams per serving

Marinated tofu is very well processed in this recipe. The outside is light and crisp and the inside is soft. If you haven't eat udon, now is your chance.

INGREDIENTS

- ½ cup of seafood sauce
- 4 tablespoons soy sauce
- 4 ounces extra-firm tofu, drained, pressed and cubed
- ¼ cup cornstarch or potato starch
- 2 tablespoons coconut oil
- 7 ounces packaged organic udon noodles
- ½ cup plus 2 tablespoons vegetable broth
- ¼ cup peanut butter
- 5 ounces baby spinach

INSTRUCTIONS

1. In a small bowl, mix hoisin and 2 tablespoons soy sauce. Add cubed tofu, toss and marinade for 30 minutes.
2. Place the corn starch on a large plate. Take out the tofu from the marinade, line it on cornstarch and throw it to cover all sides.
3. Heat the oil on a medium high heat in a large frying pan. Add tofu to hot oil and fry on all sides. Set aside.

4. Put water in a large pot and cover it. Bring to a boil and add udon. Cook for 5 minutes and drain. Set aside.
5. Add soup and peanut butter to the same saucepan and bring to a boil. Reduce heat and cook for 2 minutes, then add udon to pan. Put the sauce on the udon. Put the spinach in a pan and stir the sauce and noodles. Continue cooking on low heat for about 3 minutes until the spinach has wilted.
6. Remove from heat and split into two bowls. Place half of the tofu on each udon. Drizzle the remaining hoisin mixture from above.

DAY 25

BREAKFAST: SPICED CAULIFLOWER TEMPEH SALAD BOWL

Active Time: 20 minutes
Cook time: 15 minutes
Total Time: 35 minutes
Yield: 2 YIELD

Protein: 20 grams per serving

Baked cauliflower comes into its own with some spices added. Marinate tempeh in a slightly tangy dressing, add a little more color and taste contrast, and you'll be in power mode in no time.

INGREDIENTS

Bowl

- 1 small head of cauliflower, cut into florets
- 2 tablespoons extra virgin olive oil
- 1 teaspoon salt

- ½ teaspoon ground cumin
- ¼ teaspoon ground black pepper

Dressing

- ½ cup vegan mayonnaise
- ¼ cup unsweetened dairy-free milk
- 1 teaspoon lemon juice
- ¼ teaspoon garlic powder
- ¼ teaspoon onion powder
- ¼ teaspoon dill weed
- Pinch of salt
- Pinch of ground black pepper
- 8 ounces tempeh, sliced into ¼-inch-thick slices and then into small bite-size pieces
- 8 ounces baby spinach
- 1 small red onion, cut into bite-size pieces
- 2 carrots, cut into small matchstick pieces
- 1 yellow bell pepper, cut into bite-size pieces

INSTRUCTIONS

Cauliflower

1. Preheat the oven to 400°F.
2. Position cauliflower florets into a big bowl. Sprinkle with the oil, salt, cumin, and ¼ teaspoon pepper. Bake about 25 minutes or until you can easily pierce the cauliflower with a fork. Remove from the oven and set aside.

Dressing

3. While the cauliflower is baking, make the salad dressing. Mix the mayonnaise, milk, lemon juice, garlic and onion powders, dill weed, salt, and pinch of pepper in a small bowl. Place the tempeh in the dressing to marinate while the cauliflower is baking.

Assembly

4. Divide the spinach between two salad bowls. Make a line in the shape of an arc with each vegetable starting with the onion and continuing on with the carrots, cauliflower, and bell pepper. Remove tempeh from the marinade and add it as the final touch to the bowl. Serve with the dressing.

LUNCH: CARIBBEAN CHILI
Active Time: 30 minutes
Cook time: 1 hour
Total Time: 1 hour 30 minutes
Yield: 4 YIELD

Protein: 13 grams per serving

Treat yourself to some spicy chili with a bucketful of veggies. This recipe can be served all year round because of its warmth in the winter and its summer festive vibe.

INGREDIENTS

- 2 tablespoons coconut oil
- 1 onion, diced
- 1 green pepper, diced
- 3 Roma tomatoes, chopped
- 2 carrots, diced
- 5 ounces tomato paste
- 2 tablespoons chili powder
- 1 teaspoon salt
- 1 teaspoon ground cumin
- ½ teaspoon cinnamon

- ½ teaspoon allspice
- ½ teaspoon dried oregano
- ½ teaspoon cayenne pepper
- ¼ teaspoon garlic powder
- ¼ teaspoon garlic, minced
- ¼ teaspoon ground black pepper
- 1 oz 15 oz kidney beans, drain, rinse
- 1 corn, grain cut from cob

INSTRUCTIONS

1. Apply heat to oil in the big skillet over an average heat and add the onions and peppers. Fry for about 10-15 minutes until the onions are translucent.
2. Add tomatoes, carrots, tomato paste and 1/2 cup of water. Add spices and herbs. Bring to a boil, cover and boil for 30 minutes.
3. Add the kidney beans and corn. Boil and simmer on a low for fifteen minutes.

DINNER: SLOW COOKER VERSATILE SEITAN BALLS

Slow Cooker Size: 6 quarts

Active Time: 15 minutes

Cook time: 6 hours

Total Time: 6 hours 15 minutes

Yield: 3 cups or 34 balls

Protein: 30 grams per serving (½ cup)

These little round balls add so much flavor and texture to your hardy dishes. They make a fantastic foundation for marinara sauce submarine sandwiches, too.

INGREDIENTS

- 1½ cups vital wheat gluten
- ½ cup chickpea flour
- 1 tablespoon mushroom powder
- ½ teaspoon dried oregano
- ½ teaspoon onion powder
- ¼ teaspoon garlic powder
- ¼ teaspoon nutmeg
- ¼ teaspoon ground ginger
- ¼ teaspoon ground cloves
- ¼ teaspoon ground sage
- ½ teaspoon salt
- ½ cup tomato sauce, divided
- 1 teaspoon liquid smoke
- 1½ cups vegetable broth, divided

INSTRUCTIONS

1. Mix the gluten, flour, mushroom powder, oregano, onion and garlic powders, nutmeg, ginger, cloves, sage, and salt in a large bowl.
2. In a small bowl, add ¼ cup tomato sauce, ¼ cup water, liquid smoke, and ½ cup vegetable broth. Mix well.
3. Put a hole in the middle of the dry ingredients and pour in the tomato sauce mixture. Mix well and start to knead. Knead for 1 minute or until the dough becomes mildly elastic. You will see the dough slightly pull back as you are kneading and it will be a bit sticky. Pour remaining ¼ cup tomato sauce, 1 cup vegetable broth, and 3 cups water into the slow cooker. Stir.
4. Tear off small chunks of the dough, squeeze into a round shape, and drop into the liquid in the slow cooker. There will be forty-four balls. You can also make seventeen larger balls and cut them after cooking and cooling. Or make two logs and cut into desired shapes.

Close the lid and boil for 6 hours. They will grow in size as they cook. Check at 4 hours and see if you like the texture. They will become firmer as they sit in the refrigerator.
5. Remove from the pot and let cool. Serve and Enjoy

DAY 26

BREAKFAST: BROCCOLI VEGETABLE DIPPER
Active time: 10 minutes
Cook Time: 25 minutes
Total time: 35 minutes
Yield: 6 YIELD

Protein: 6 grams per serving (2 patties)

Please enjoy vegetables. These dippers are small putties that can be picked up with your finger. Eat as it is or soak it in your favorite sauce. Party food!

INGREDIENTS:

- ¾Lentils
- 2 cups broccoli florets, fresh
- 1 tbsp chia seed
- Shredded carrots in cup
- ¼ teaspoon garlic powder
- ¼ teaspoon parsley
- 1/2 teaspoon salt
- ¼ teaspoon ground black pepper
- ¼ teaspoon onion powder
- ¼ teaspoon dried oregano
- ¼ 1 teaspoon of dried basil

- ¾ cup bread crumbs, split
- 1 tbsp extra virgin olive oil

INSTRUCTIONS:

1. Rinse the lentils and drain. Put the lentils in a medium to large pot. ½Pour a cup of water. Bring the pot over high heat to a boil. When the water boils, lower it to medium and cook for 20 minutes or until the lentils are soft. All water must be absorbed. Set aside.
2. In the meantime, add water to a medium-sized pan , boil and add the broccoli while steam in boiling water for 10 minutes. Remove from the steamer and set aside.
3. Mix the ground chia seeds with 3 tablespoons of water in a small bowl.
4. Put all ingredients except the crumbs in the cup into the food processor. It has a friable texture and is processed until it binds well. Divide the mixture into 12 pieces. Roll each piece into a ball and flatten it on the putty. Coat each putty on both sides with the remaining crumbs.
5. Heat the oil to medium height in a medium frying pan and burn the putty on both sides for 3 minutes.
6. Serve dairy-free chipotle mayonnaise or other favorite spicy dip sauce.

LUNCH: CHOCOLATE STRAWBERRY CHIA SEED PUDDING

Active time: 15 minutes

Chill time: 4 hours

Total time: 4 hours 15 minutes

Yield: 2 YIELD

Protein: 16 grams per serving

Get your fruit and protein with this breakfast in run. Make this pudding recipe the night before and prepare a breakfast stuffed with simple fruits. **ACTIVE TIME** is only a few minutes.

INGREDIENTS:

- 1 cup milk without dairy
- ⅓ Cup date
- ½Cup strawberries (for garnish, additional)
- 2 tablespoons cocoa powder
- 1/2 teaspoon vanilla essence
- ¼Cup Ground Chia Seed
- 3 tablespoons of raw
- 2 tablespoons maple syrup
- For shaving chocolate and garnish (optional)

INSTRUCTIONS:

1. Add milk and date to the blender. Mix until smooth. Add strawberries, cocoa powder, vanilla, chia seeds, hemp seeds and maple syrup. Mix well. Pour into two bowls and refrigerate for at least 4 hours.
2. If necessary, decorate the cut chocolate and strawberries.

DINNER: SLOW COOKER MAPLE BREAKFAST LINKS

Slow Cooker Size: 6 quarts
Active Time: 20 minutes
Cook time: 6 hours
Total Time: 6 hours 20 minutes
Yield: 4 cups or 32 small links

Protein: 22½ grams per serving

These tender and sweet links can be sliced for multiple recipes. Freeze the seitan for a quick meal anytime.

INGREDIENTS

- 2 cups vegetable broth
- 1½ cups vital wheat gluten
- ½ cup chickpea flour
- 2 teaspoons ground sage, divided
- ¼ teaspoon onion powder
- ¼ teaspoon garlic powder
- 1 teaspoon salt
- ¼ cup tomato sauce
- 2 tablespoons maple syrup
- 2 tablespoons ketchup
- 1 teaspoon coconut oil

INSTRUCTIONS

1. Put the broth and 2 cups water in slow cooker. Turn to low. Add the gluten, flour, sage, onion powder, garlic powder, and salt to a large bowl. Mix well.
2. In a separate small bowl, add ½ cup water, tomato sauce, maple syrup, ketchup, and oil. Mix well.
3. Put a hole in the middle of dry mixture and pour in the tomato sauce mixture. Start to stir. This comes together quickly. Squeeze in one hand and let it go through your fingers about 10 times. Start to knead in the bowl. It is a wet mixture but will start to become elastic. Knead for about 3 minutes for a softer and tender breakfast link. The longer you knead, the more elastic it becomes. I keep it all in the bowl for kneading. It is much easier to clean up.

4. Pinch off small chunks and then roll between the palms of your hands, pretty quickly, back and forth. This will make thirty-two small links. You really can't form pretty links, but they will work fine in any recipe you make. Alternatively, you can make fifteen larger links. The larger size would change each link to 15 grams protein.
5. Place the links in the liquid in the slow cooker. Cover and cook on low for 6 hours. They will grow in size as they cook.
6. Remove from the slow cooker and let cool. Refrigerate for up to 5 days and use as needed. They freeze really well, with or without their liquid.

DAY 27

BREAKFAST: LOADED SWEET POTATO BURRITOS
Active Time: 15 minutes
Cook time: 20 minutes
Total Time: 35 minutes
Yield: 6 YIELD

Protein: 19 grams per serving

The spicy and sweet contrast in these burritos really hits the spot. This is an updated classic, and you can fill up your tortillas as full as you like.

INGREDIENTS

- 1 tablespoon coconut oil
- 1 sweet potato, peeled and diced
- 8 ounces mushrooms, sliced

- ¾ cup diced red onion
- ¾ cup diced red bell pepper
- 1½ cups Steamed Seitan Smoky Nuggets
- 1½ teaspoons chili powder
- ½ teaspoon garlic powder
- ¼ teaspoon ground cumin
- 2 cups baby spinach, torn small
- 6 whole wheat or sprouted grain tortillas

INSTRUCTIONS

1. using an average heat, heat up oil with a huge skillet. Add the sweet potato, mushrooms, onion, and bell pepper. Sauté for 15 minutes. Add the seitan, chili powder, garlic powder, and cumin, and cook for 5 more minutes. Add the spinach and cook just a minute or so until wilted.
2. If the tortillas are stiff, such as sprouted grain, then you can warm them in a microwave for 10 to 15 seconds. This will make them easier to roll.
3. Spoon about 1 cup of sweet potato mixture down the center of each tortilla. Roll up. Cut in half for easier handling.

LUNCH: THIN SLICES AND CRUMBLES SLOW COOKER
Active Time: 10 minutes
Cook time: 6 hours
Total Time: 6 hours 10 minutes
Yield: 4 YIELD

Protein: 31 grams per serving (½ cup)

One large oval log is a perfect shape for slicing. You have the option of cutting the log into nuggets or you can crumble it. This versatility makes this seitan a go-to for a multitude of recipes.

INGREDIENTS

- 1¼ cups vital wheat gluten
- ¼ cup chickpea flour
- 1 tablespoon mushroom powder
- 2 tablespoon nutritional yeast
- ½ teaspoon ground sage
- ½ teaspoon salt
- ¼ teaspoon garlic powder
- ¼ teaspoon onion powder
- ¾ cup tomato sauce
- 1 tablespoon tomato paste
- 2 cups vegetable broth
- ¼ cup tomato sauce

INSTRUCTIONS

1. Add the gluten, flour, mushroom powder, nutritional yeast, sage, salt, and garlic and onion powders to a large bowl.
2. Mix tomato sauce, tomato paste, and ¼ cup plus 1 tablespoon water in a small bowl. Put both the wet mixture and dry together
3. Mix and then knead for about 2 to 3 minutes or until mildly elastic. You will see the dough slightly pull back as you are kneading and it will be a bit sticky. Shape the seitan into a log.
4. Pour 1 cup water, the vegetable broth, and tomato sauce into a 2½- to 3-quart slow cooker. Place the log in the slow cooker or roll loosely in cloth and tie each end with cotton string. It does expand when cooking, so you shouldn't roll it tight. If you don't care that the outside is a bit lumpier after being cooked, then don't bother to roll in cloth. Cover slow cooker and turn to low. Cook on low for 6 hours.

5. Remove the log from the liquid and place aside to cool. Serve and keep in the refrigerator. It can also be frozen for 4 months.

DINNER: ACADIAN BLACK BEANS AND RICE
Active Time: 5 minutes
Cook time: 40 minutes
Total Time: 45 minutes
Yield: 6 YIELD

Protein: 16 grams per serving

Here's an updated version of that Southern classic, red beans and rice. This version is made with a variety of spices popular in Cajun country.

INGREDIENTS

- 1½ cups brown rice
- 3½ cups low sodium vegetable broth
- 1 tablespoon extra virgin olive oil
- ½ yellow onion, chopped
- 1 green bell pepper, chopped
- 2 15-ounce cans black beans, drained and rinsed
- 1 clove garlic, finely chopped
- ¼ cup diced tomatoes
- 1 teaspoon parsley
- 1 teaspoon garlic powder
- 1 teaspoon onion powder
- 1 teaspoon thyme
- 1 teaspoon oregano
- ½ teaspoon cayenne pepper
- ¼ teaspoon ground black pepper

- 1 teaspoon salt

INSTRUCTIONS

1. Cook the brown rice by any method you choose. I use a rice cooker. Cook the rice with vegetable broth for this recipe.
2. using a big Skillet heat up oil to an average heat and then add the onion and bell pepper. Sauté until the onion becomes transparent, about 10 minutes. Minus the rice, add every other ingredient to the large skillet with the onion and bell pepper. Cook for 10 minutes. Add the rice and heat through.

DAY 28

BREAKFAST: APRICOT PISTACHIO ENERGY SQUARES

Active Time: 15 minutes
Cook time: 10 minutes
Refrigerator Time: 30 minutes
Total Time: 55 minutes
Yield: 16 squares

Protein: 8 grams per serving (2 squares)

Every good flavor you can think of is in these perfect little squares. Besides heavenly apricot and dates, you have the option of drizzling chocolate over the top.

INGREDIENTS

- 1½ cups pitted dates, chopped
- 1 cup dried apricots, chopped
- 1 cup cashews, chopped

- ½ cup old-fashioned oats
- ½ cup pistachios
- 3 tablespoons cashew butter
- 2 tablespoons ground ginger
- ⅓ cup brown rice syrup
- 2 tablespoons maple syrup
- 1 teaspoon vanilla extract
- ¼ cup dairy-free chocolate chips (optional)

INSTRUCTIONS

1. Position an 8 "square baking platter with baking parchment and come up about 3 inches on opposite sides. This will act as a handle to remove the squares from the dish.
2. Add the dates, apricots, cashews, oats, and pistachios to a large bowl. Mix in the cashew butter and ground ginger and combine as well as you can. You can use your fingers to help blend it all together.
3. In a small saucepan, add the brown rice syrup, maple syrup, and vanilla. Bring to a boil and continue boiling until it reaches the hard ball stage, 260°F, on a candy thermometer. Quickly add to the date mixture and mix well. Pour into the prepared dish and press firmly and evenly into all edges and corners. Refrigerate at least 30 minutes.
4. Grab the "handles" of the parchment paper and lift out of the dish. Place on a cutting sheet and slice into sixteen squares.
5. If desired, melt the chocolate chips in a microwave or in a small saucepan. Drizzle back and forth over the bars.

LUNCH: RAINBOW VEGGIE PROTEIN PINWHEELS
Active time: 20 minutes
Total time: 20 minutes
Yield: 6 YIELD

Protein: 9g per serving (2 windmills)

Spread vegetables on a bed of hummus and crushed tempe and wrap everything in a perfect holder, a green spinach tortilla. Even the most likes and dislikes will want to eat.

INGREDIENTS:

- ¼Cup Hummus
- ¼Cup tempe, crushed with a food processor
- Two large spinach tortillas
- Red pepper sliced cup
- ¼ cup sliced yellow pepper
- 1 carrot, sliced
- Very thin sliced cup of purple cabbage

INSTRUCTIONS:
1. Mix hummus and tempeh.
2. Put the tortilla. Spread the hummus mixture in a thin layer over the surface of each tortilla and stop 1 inch from the edge. Place a thin strip of each of the four vegetables next to the hummus mixture.
3. Roll each tortilla firmly and cut it sideways into a windmill. You can use nail pic branches if needed, but Hummus will help them stick at the edges.

DINNER: EDAMAME AND BROCCOLI RICE BOWL
Active Time: 20 minutes
Cook time: 30 minutes
Total Time: 50 minutes
Yield: 2 YIELD

Protein: 20 grams per serving
Tahini sauce pulls this rice-based bowl all together. Each vegetable can stand on its own, but when they mingle with each other, the result is memorable.

INGREDIENTS
Bowl

- ½ cup broccoli florets
- ½ cup edamame, frozen
- ¼ teaspoon salt
- ¼ cup peas, frozen or fresh
- ½ cup chopped yellow bell pepper

Tahini Sauce

- ¼ cup tahini
- 1 tablespoon lemon juice
- 1 tablespoon maple syrup
- 1 tablespoon tamari

To Assemble

- 2 cups jasmine rice, cooked
- ¼ cup sunflower seed kernels
- ¼ cup raisins

INSTRUCTIONS
Bowl
1. Add water to a medium-sized pan, boil and add the broccoli

while steaming in boiling water for 10 minutes. Remove from the steamer and set aside.

2. Bring 2 cups water to a boil in a small saucepan and add the edamame and salt. Boil for 5 minutes, adding the peas during the last minute. Drain and set aside.

3. Meanwhile, add 2 tablespoons water to a small skillet and heat over medium-high heat. Sauté for 10 minutes after you have added the pepper bell. Remove from the heat and set aside.

Tahini Sauce

4. Add all the ingredients plus 5 tablespoons water to a small bowl and blend until smooth.

Assembly

5. Add the rice to the bottom of each bowl. Divide the remaining items in half and add onto the rice in a pinwheel fashion, making sure that the greens don't touch each other for a more pleasing design.

6. Serve with the tahini sauce.

DAY 29

BREAKFAST: CRUNCHY NUTS AND SEEDS PROTEIN BARS

Active Time: 15 minutes
Refrigerator Time: 30 minutes
Total Time: 45 minutes
Yield: 16 bars
Protein: 9 grams per serving (1 bar)

A little miracle happens after these bars cool. They turn into a caramel-like bar that gives satisfaction to no end. Chocolaty and chewy!

INGREDIENTS

- 2 cups chickpea flour
- 1 cup plus 2 tablespoons almond flour
- 2 tablespoons flaxseed meal
- 1 cup dairy-free milk
- 1 cup cashew butter
- ½ cup maple syrup
- ½ cup slivered almonds
- ½ cup dried cranberries
- ¼ cup sunflower seed kernels
- ½ cup dairy-free chocolate chips, melted

INSTRUCTIONS

1. Cover square baking bowl with parchment paper and come up about 3 inches on opposite sides. This will act as a handle to remove the bars from the dish.
2. Combine the flours and flaxseed meal in a large bowl and mix well. With a heavy wooden spoon, mix in the milk, cashew butter, maple syrup, almonds, cranberries, and sunflower seeds. Lastly, mix in the melted chocolate. Add the batter to the prepared dish and press firmly into all corners and as evenly as possible. Refrigerate for at least 30 minutes.
3. Grab the "handles" of the parchment paper and lift out of the dish. Place on a cutting sheet and slice into sixteen bars.

LUNCH: BLUEBERRY TOFU PANCAKE

Active time: 10 minutes
COOK TIME: 10 minutes
Total time: 20 minutes
Yield: 4 YIELD

Protein: 17 grams per serving (3 pancakes)

Eating a bit of sweets in the morning is fine, especially when eating pancakes full of tofu and oats.

INGREDIENTS

- 2 tablespoons flax seed meal
- 8 oz firm tofu, drained and pressed
- ½ cup of traditional oats
- 1¼ cup milk without dairy
- 1 cup general purpose flour
- 3 tablespoons of coconut sugar
- 1 teaspoon of vanilla essence
- 1 teaspoon baking powder
- 1 tsp cinnamon
- 1/2 teaspoon salt
- 1/2 teaspoon and 1 tablespoon extra virgin olive oil, split
- ¼Cup maple syrup for serving
- ½ cup frozen blueberries, thaw, split

INSTRUCTIONS

1. Mix flax seed meal with 6 tablespoons of water and save.
2. Add all ingredients except the blueberries and a tablespoon of oil to the food processor and mix well. Use the quick pulse button to blend 1/4 cup blueberries.
3. Apply heat to oil in a frying pan and add ¼ cup of pancake dough to the center of the pan. When whisking one side, turn over and cook until golden. Continue until all batters are gone.
4. Sprinkle the maple syrup and the remaining ¼ cup of blueberries on top.

DINNER: WHITE BEAN STEW WITH CHIPOTLE LINKS
Active Time: 15 minutes
Soaking Time: 8 hours
Cook time: 2 hours 20 minutes
Total Time: 10 hours 35 minutes

Protein: 27 grams per serving

Yield: 6 YIELD
This stew is an all-time favorite. It has fresh carrots and corn off the cob, and the plant-based chipotle links give it a sensational taste and texture.

INGREDIENTS

- 1 pound navy beans
- 1 cup Steamed Seitan Chipotle
- 2 tablespoons extra virgin olive oil
- ½ cup diced onion
- 2 carrots, peeled and chopped
- 2 cloves garlic, finely diced
- 2 15-ounce cans fire-roasted tomatoes
- 2 cobs of corn, kernels cut from the cob
- 1 cup vegetable broth
- 1 teaspoon basil
- 1 teaspoon hot sauce, such as Tabasco (omit if you don't like spicy; you can put it on the table instead)

INSTRUCTIONS
The Night Before Cooking
1. Place the beans in a big pot and cover with water. Swallow your hand in the water, and pick up some floating beans or not looking good. Drain the beans. Place the beans back in the large pot. Fill

about 4 inches above the beans with water. Let it soak up overnight on the counter.

The 2nd day

Drain the beans and cover them with 2 to 3 cm of fresh water. Cover and add to a boil. Turn the heat down to low medium and boil for around 11/2 to 2 hours, partially covered. Stir a few times during the **COOK TIME**, however ensure that the temperature remains in a decent simmer and that the beans are filled with water. When you can flatten one with your fingers the beans are finished.

3. When the beans are almost done, brown the seitan links on all sides. Remove from the pan and cut into about ¾-inch pieces.

4. With a big Skillet start heating over a low heat, add oil and add the chopped onion and carrots and sauté for 10 minutes. Add the garlic and cook for 1 minute.

To Finish

5. Remove water from beans and put back in the big pot. Now add and boil the tomatoes for ten minutes. It will be soupy. Add the corn, broth, basil, and hot sauce and bring to a boil. Turn down the heat and simmer another 10 minutes.

DAY 30

BREAKFAST: CHOCOLATE CHIP BANANA BREAD PROTEIN COOKIES

Active Time: 15 minutes

Cook time: 15 minutes

Total Time: 30 minutes

Yield: 12 YIELD

Protein: 6 grams per serving (2 cookies)

These protein-rich cookies have a high fiber content that fills you up and helps keep you feeling satisfied. They taste delicious, too!

INGREDIENTS

- 2 tablespoons of chia seed or ground chia seed
- 1 cup whole wheat flour
- ½ cup almond flour
- ½ cup flaxseed meal
- 2 tablespoons protein powder
- ½ teaspoon baking soda
- ½ teaspoon salt
- ¾ cup dairy-free butter
- ⅔ cup coconut sugar
- ⅓ cup organic light brown sugar, packed
- 1 teaspoon vanilla extract
- ½ cup banana, mashed (1 medium banana)
- 1 cup dairy-free chocolate chips

INSTRUCTIONS

1. Preheat the oven to 350°F. Cut parchment paper on a baking sheet to match. put aside
2. Mix the chia seeds with 6 tablespoons water and set aside.
3. Add both flours, the flaxseed, protein powder, baking soda, and salt to a large bowl. Set aside.
4. Add butter and both sugars to the bowl of a stand mixer. Mix on medium speed for 5 minutes. Switch off beater then add mixture of chia seeds, cinnamon, and banana to cook. Mix well to low velocity. Add the dry ingredients, and start to mix until just combined. Clear the chocolate chips from mixing bowl and fold.

5. Place heaping tablespoons on a cookie sheet 2 inches apart and flatten with the bottom of a glass to about ½ inch thick. Bake for 12 minutes.
6. Cool on a wire rack.

LUNCH: SEITAN NUGGETS ROTELLE

Active Time: 10 minutes
Cook time: 20 minutes
Total Time: 30 minutes
Yield: 6 YIELD

Protein: 20 grams per serving

It's always a good thing when you can get a family meal on the table in under 30 minutes, especially when you're serving comfort food to the max.

INGREDIENTS

- 3 cups rotelle pasta
- 1 tablespoon extra virgin olive oil
- ½ cup chopped onion
- 2 cups Steamed Seitan Smoky Nuggets, cut into bite-size pieces if necessary
- 2 cloves garlic, finely chopped
- 1 15-ounce can diced tomatoes
- ½ teaspoon Italian seasoning
- ½ teaspoon salt
- ¼ teaspoon ground black pepper

- Scallions, for garnish (optional)

INSTRUCTIONS

1. Cook rotelle according to directions on the package.
2. Meanwhile, heat the oil in a large skillet over medium-high heat. Add the onion and seitan and sauté for 10 minutes until the onion is translucent. Ensure you cook for about one minute after adding the garlic. Add the diced tomatoes, Italian seasoning, salt, and pepper. Bring to a boil and turn to cook for 5 minutes. Add the cooked rotelle. Heat through for 5 minutes.
3. If you'd like, garnish with the scallions.

DINNER: BLACK BEAN AND LENTIL SUPER BURRITOS SLOW COOKED

Active Time: 15 minutes

Cook time: 8 hours

Total Time: 8 hours 15 minutes

Yield: 6 YIELD

Protein: 21 grams per serving (2 burritos)

These super easy burritos are spicy with lots of texture. The addition of avocados and black olives makes for a hearty meal.

INGREDIENTS

- 2 cans, 15ounce diced tomatoes
- ¼ cup salsa
- 2 cans, 15ounce black beans that is drained and rinsed
- 1 cup brown rice
- ½ cup corn, fresh, frozen, or canned
- 2 tablespoons taco seasoning
- 1 teaspoon ground cumin

- 1 teaspoon salt
- 2 peppers (chipotle) in adobo sauce, finely chopped
- 2½ cups vegetable broth
- ½ cup lentils
- 12 whole wheat tortillas
- Additional toppings, such as more salsa, avocado or guacamole, and black olives

INSTRUCTIONS

1. In a slow cooker add the tomatoes, lettuce, peppers, peas, corn, taco seasoning, cumin, butter, chipotles and broth. Stir and hide. Boil slowly for 8 hours, or for about 4 hours if you want it quicker.
2. Over the last 40 minutes of cooking substitute the lentils. Continue to cook until the lentils get tender. Without water the rice stays dry and soft. That is the filling out.
4. Lay the tortillas out and place the filling on each tortilla about 1/3 to 1/2 cup (for a very large burrito). Stretch the filling out through the tortilla core. Fold each end approximately 11/2 inches above the edge of the beans. Then turn the tortilla's long surface upwards. Move straight ahead once you have that plan that you'd like to use on these. 4. Stack up on more salsa, mango, or guacamole, and eat black olives.

Plant-Based High Protein Cookbook

130+ Easy and Fast Vegan and Vegetarian Protein Recipes for Muscle Growth and Energy Boost
Nutritional Guide for Athletes!

MANUEL MILLER

INTRODUCTION TO PLANT-BASED HIGH PROTEIN

Plant foods are generally classified as fruits, vegetables, legumes, grains, nuts, and seeds. Derived products such as bread, pasta, breakfast cereals, cooked and fermented vegetables and legumes, fruit purees, juices and jams, derived ingredients such as oil, sugar, some herbs and spices from oily seeds

What distinguishes them from animal foods is that their fiber fraction is made up of resistant compounds consisting mainly of cellulose, hemicellulose, pectin, and / or resistant starch. Among cereal products, legumes, cereals / pseudocereals, and nuts / seed are characterized by high carbohydrate, protein, and lipid content, respectively. In addition to fiber, all plant-based foods have macro (proteins, lipids, carbohydrates), micros (minerals, trace elements, vitamins), and phytonutrients (polyphenols, carotenoids, etc.). Each of them helps plants survive in their environment and renew themselves.

By definition, a bioactive compound has a biological effect in a human organism, tissue, or cell, and is likely to have a prophylactic effect on pathophysiological processes. Thus, in plant-based foods, all compounds or nutrients are potentially biologically active in the human body, but their protective effects depend on the health or physiological condition, the degree of food processing, and other factors in the food. The matrix depends on several factors, such as the presence of the compound, and consumption. Even anti nutritional factors such as phytate have potential protective effects, highlighting the dual nature of bioactive compounds in plants. In addition, biologically active compounds are rarely protected by themselves, but are synergistic with other compounds. This is highlighted by compounds with properties related to antioxidants and lipophilicity.

Plant-based foods can be eaten raw, but most are processed to be safe, edible, and / or more palatable, especially for grain-based foods. Processing can range from minimal, such as soaking legume seeds, to very dramatic, such as extruding white flour.

Processing also includes blending vegetable foods with ingredients such as fats and cooking agents. In all cases, the potential package of the biologically active compound is clearly modified in clearly different ways. In particular, when refining removes most of the minerals and vitamins in cereal products.

The protein has become one of the favorite nutrients today. It is quite common to hear comments like: "I have to eat some protein", "I did not eat enough protein today" or "Do you want to add protein to your salad?" But it is also true that every day we move away from animal proteins, and we begin to discover ingredients of plant origin rich in this nutrient.

In the 1980s and 1990s, people considered fat to be bad and carbohydrates to be good. The food pyramid told us to base our diets on carbohydrates . In the early 2000s, we realized that overconsumption of carbohydrates, specifically refined carbohydrates, was not so good for us.
Today we know that diets high in refined carbohydrates increase the risk of type 2 diabetes , as well as heart disease. And since we still have doubts about whether fats are good or bad, protein seems like the best substitute for carbohydrates. In addition, plant-based food, such as vegetarian and vegan , are also trending. This is due to various factors such as the sustainability of the food supply, especially for a growing population, animal treatment and human health.

Humans need 20 amino acids to make proteins. Of those 20 amino acids, nine are essential , which means that the human body cannot produce them, so we have to get them from food. Plants contain all the essential amino acids, but the proportions are lower, which is why they are known as incomplete proteins . The biggest myth about protein consumption is that certain plant foods lack amino acids, and these are only available in plant-based foods.

We always talk about food balance, so instead of focusing on just one nutrient, it's important to analyze its benefits and harms . For example, legumes, seeds, and nuts are high in protein and also provide fiber , vitamin E, and protective phytochemicals. To choose the best source of protein, you must consider what other nutrients accompany it.

Lately flexitarianism has become fashionable, a word that mixes flexible and vegetarianism. The goal is to eat plant-based foods and be a vegetarian. The idea is to see meat as a secondary ingredient, which adds flavor, texture and interest. Flexitarianism is very much like some of the healthiest diets in the world , including the Mediterranean diet and traditional Asian cuisine.

HOW MUCH PROTEIN DOES THE BODY NEED?

The protein requirement in humans depends on the genetic requirements, age, stress, physical activity and protein quality of the food. This can therefore vary greatly depending on the constitution. Science has calculated that the minimum protein requirement is around 0.34g per kg body weight. The DGE recommends 56g of protein per day for a man weighing approximately 70 kg. This corresponds to 0.8g per kg of body weight.

The recommended amount I would say of protein is 0.8 grams per kilogram of body weight. If we see protein intake as a percentage of total calories, the recommendation is that between 10% -35% of calories are protein.

This safety cushion compared to the minimum requirement also makes sense, since both the biological value in the protein varies and the ability of the digestive tract to assimilate is different for each person. For a recreational athlete, this amount should be absolutely sufficient.

In competitive sports, the protein requirement can grow up to 2g per kg. This affects above all endurance athletes. There are now excellent vegetable protein powders in raw food quality.

It is interesting that far too much protein is now consumed in western cultures, especially when consuming animal products. Excessive protein consumption can strain the kidneys and lead to diseases such as gout (protein breakdown products are deposited in the joints).

One of the most common questions that vegans are asked is surely about an adequate protein supply. Proteins are found in practically all plant foods. The following list represents a small selection of foods that are characterized, among other things, by a high protein content; all without animal fats and animal protein and above all without animal suffering. All groceries are not only to be found in almost every supermarket and most discounters, but are also inexpensive, tasty and versatile.

1. Beans
Black, white, kidney, broad or pinto beans - as large as the number of different types of beans is, their use is varied. Whether in chili sin carne, in salads, wraps and burritos or as an antipasti on crostini's, as a warm puree or as a dip or something unusual but unusually delicious in chocolate-sweet brownies - there are no limits to the imagination when vegan cooking and baking with beans.

2. Tofu
Tofu can be grilled, fried and baked marinated; it can be processed whole or crumbled and in pureed form it offers an ideal basis for delicious sauces, smoothies and creams. When smoked or refined with tomatoes, olives or herbs, it is suitable as a bread topping. Because tofu, which can be found in the form of cut-resistant versions up to silk tofu depending on the water content, accepts every aroma, it is suitable for many recipes - from spicy-spicy to sweet.

3. Nuts

There is a wide range of different nuts and kernels, which are botanically not nuts, but are colloquially counted among them (examples: cashews, Brazil nuts, peanuts). They can all be used in a variety of ways and are suitable, for example, for the production of nut butter, vegetable milk and vegan "cheese variants".
They are also pure or seasoned a quick and healthy snack.

4. Tempeh
Tempeh is not as well known as tofu, but it is just as versatile. Tempeh is made from whole cooked and fermented soybeans that are formed into a solid, slightly nutty-tasting block. Just like tofu, tempeh can take on any taste and can be grilled, fried and baked. Tempeh goes well with pasta and vegetable dishes, pizza and sandwiches. The form of manufacture ensures a high protein and fiber content and good bioavailability of proteins and minerals.

5. Chickpeas
Chickpeas are very versatile legumes. They are characterized by a high proportion of the essential amino acid lysine. They go well with salads, wraps and stews. The crushed beans can be used to make patties and pureed together with sesame paste hummus.

6. Broccoli
Low calorie, rich in vitamins K and C and a good source of protein. Steamed broccoli is well suited for pasta and pan dishes, but also for salads. It goes well with soups both whole and pureed.

7. Quinoa
The pseudograin Quinoa can be used in a similar way to rice. Quinoa is suitable as a side dish, can be mixed with vegetables and provides a good basis for salads when cold. Quinoa can be used to make patties and it also works well in baked goods. The pseudo-cereal, rich in iron and folic acid, is also a delight when prepared sweetly.

8. Lentils
Because of their shorter soaking and cooking times than beans or

peas, these protein-rich legumes are also suitable for spontaneous people. Lentil dishes are classic in Germany in the form of stews and soups. But cooked lentils are also suitable cold for salads or patties and they are very popular in healthy, Mexican-style fast food such as tacos or burritos.

9. Potato
Potatoes are usually associated with a high carbohydrate content. These relatively low-calorie and vitamin C-rich tubers also contain proteins. The protein quality, i.e. its usability and its amino acid composition, is very high. The protein of the potato has a high biological value, much higher than that of other frequently consumed plants.

10. Oats
Cereals are generally characterized by a good protein content, including oats. The oatmeal is a good basis for any cereal or cereal. The combination with protein-rich plant drinks also increases the biological value here. But a slightly nutty-tasting plant drink can also be made from oats themselves. Oatmeal also gives patties and sweet baked goods the necessary bite.

CHAPTER ONE
FOODS TO AVOID

This is a diet that focuses on consuming food in the most natural way. This means that heavily processed foods are excluded.

When buying groceries, focus on fresh foods, and when buying labeled foods, aim for items with as few ingredients as possible.

Foods to avoid
Fast food: French fries, cheeseburgers, hot dogs, chicken nuggets, etc.
Added sugar and sweets: table sugar, soda, juice, pastries, cookies, candy, sweet tea, sugared cereals, etc.
Refined grains: white rice, white pasta, white bread, bagels, etc.
Convenient packaged foods: chips, crackers, cereal bars, frozen dinners, etc.
Food for processed vegans: plant-derived meats such as tofa key, fake cheese, vegan butter
Artificial sweeteners: Equal, Splenda, Sweet'N Low, etc.
Processed animal products: bacon, lunch meat, sausage, beef jerky, etc.

Interesting thing: Eating plants is a great way to get enough protein (and enough calories, vitamins and minerals, healthy fats and fiber).

To do this, simply eat various legumes, grains, nuts, seeds, vegetables and fruits. That way, you can get all the right nutrients without using any dietary cholesterol, and in fact leave no room for animal food. Animal products may seem like an easy way to inject protein and iron, but for balance, they are not an absolutely necessary part of our diet.

THE PLANT BASED ATHLETE GETTING STARTED

Regardless of your eating style, carbohydrates are the key to promoting workouts. You will be familiar with carbohydrate-rich plant foods such as grains, potatoes, and fruits. It's not difficult to get enough carbs during a plant-based diet! Occasionally, all the fibers of a vegetable food can quickly fill up, and it's safe to eat refined cereals such as white pasta and white rice.

Many of us are trained to believe that protein from meat, dairy and eggs is needed to maintain strong muscle and bone. In fact, plant foods can provide all the necessary amino acids and proteins! Plant foods rich in protein include soy foods such as beans, lentils, nuts, tofu and tempeh.

Another concern about a plant-based diet as an athlete is getting enough calories. While it is true that vegetables have low calories, the botanical kingdom is rich in calories such as nuts, seeds, avocados and olives. "Nuts and seeds, nuts and seed butter are important for athletes.

"Try to cook as much as possible, but do not avoid packaged vegan food, frozen dinners, or restaurant meals, as they can help fill daily vegan athlete plates." Additional boosts during.

In addition to macronutrients (carbohydrates, proteins, fats), athletes also need to be aware of certain micronutrients (vitamin and minerals). "Iron should be in the heart of all athletes, especially plant-based vegan athletes. Fortunately, many vegetable foods contain iron and their absorption in combination with vitamin C-containing foods This combination occurs naturally: burritos salsa, falafel sandwich tomatoes, tofu scrambled peppers.

This is a nutrient that women of child-bearing age (or menstruating men) should be aware of, as women need more iron than men.

How can athletes start a plant-based diet
Think alternatives, not exclusions. Replace the meat with tofu, tempe, beans and lentils. Replace dairy-based milk, cheese and yogurt with fortified plant-based versions of these foods. Hope you have already eaten a variety of colorful vegetables and fruits, but if not, aim to add at least two different colored produce to every meal. The colors of vegetables and fruits represent a variety of nutrients that are essential for nutrition and recovery.

You also need to make some additions with the replacement. I love adding freshly baked tofu to pasta to increase the protein in my carbohydrate-based diet. In addition, try pasta based on legumes to get even more energized. Adding peanut butter to a smoothie adds protein, fat, and calories. Salad and wrap avocados are another great way to add fat, calories and taste to plant-based diets. And don't forget that you can cook with oil such as olive oil. Just because you eat on a plant basis doesn't mean you need to start overly restricting certain foods.

Looking for a specific idea for a plant-based diet or snack? "The bean dip is very good! It's tasty, easy and fast calories and protein. You can eat them with fresh vegetables, sandwiches, spoons and sauces-unlimited applications and more than hummus. There is a regular soak of white beans and black beans. "

Enjoy it, try different recipes and enjoy the taste and benefits of plant based meals!

HOW A PLANT BASED HIGH PROTEIN DIET CAN BOAST YOUR HEALTH

A plant-based totally food regimen is greater economical, in particular if you devour in-season and devour nearby produce. Check out some of these health benefits of going getting plant-powered, and start consuming extra flora this week. By filling your plate up with the good stuff, there's less room for the acidic animal ingredients that go away you sluggish and tired.

1. Lower Blood Pressure

Most humans living a plant-based food plan robotically have decrease blood strain due to a higher intake of potassium-rich meals. Potassium allows decrease blood pressure that leads to strain and anxiety. Most all complete grains, legumes, nuts, seeds, and all fruits and vegetables contain excessive quantities of potassium and Vitamin B6 (which also helps decrease blood stress). Meat and maximum all animal meals include little to no potassium and in reality improve blood pressure and cholesterol.

2. Lower Cholesterol

Speaking of lower cholesterol, it's one of the main benefits you'll receive from embracing plant-primarily based meals. Most people don't recognise that flowers incorporate NO cholesterol, even saturated sources like coconut and cacao. While you need to balance your fats consumption no matter in case you're vegan or not, a plant-based totally weight loss program is one of the handiest ways to decrease cholesterol. Consider this: one egg has twice the quantity of cholesterol as a fast meals hamburger and fish contains nearly or even greater ldl cholesterol than meat or poultry, depending on the sort you consume. Plant foods like vegetables, culmination, entire grains, nuts, and seeds can simply decrease fees of cholesterol and coronary heart disease. For more on looking after your ldl cholesterol, check out these tremendous tips to take care of your cholesterol on a vegan weight loss plan.

3. Better Blood Sugar

The variety one manner to combat excessive blood sugar is to devour greater fiber. Its slows down absorption of sugars within the blood move and as a end result can help improve how hungry you are all day long, not to say balance your cortisol tiers that motive strain. Animal meals had been discovered to raise blood sugar, despite the myth that they assist combat it.

4. Lower Rates of Cancer

A low fat, entire ingredients plant-based totally diet is the quantity one manner to enhance your probabilities at heading off cancer risks (whilst also averting smoking and alcohol, of course). Animal ingredients had been connected to most cancers, especially colon and breast most cancers.

5. Weight Management

If you're consuming an entire meals, plant-based weight loss plan (especially one that's low in fat and processed sugars), you're probable to enjoy higher weight management. A meals high in raw, smooth whole foods may improve your possibilities at losing weight even extra, despite the fact that cooked ingredients may help with nutrient absorption. Weight loss (if that's what you need health-wise) can naturally occur while you consume greater fiber, vitamins, and minerals than you do animal fat and proteins. Within two weeks of a plant-based weight loss program, maximum humans lose five kilos without going hungry or feeling deprived.

CHAPTER TWO
PLANT-BASED PROTEIN RECIPE

SEITAN MAPLE LINKS BREAKFAST SANDWICH

Active time: 15 minutes
Cook Time: 20 minutes
Total time: 35 minutes
Yield: 2 YIELD

Protein: 34 grams per serving

The soft Seitan rink from the slow cooker is the star of this hearty and savory breakfast.

INGREDIENTS

- 1 tbsp extra virgin olive oil
- 8 oz mushrooms, sliced
- 1 tablespoon dairy-free butter
- 1 cup slow cooker maple breakfast link
- 2 English muffins, sliced
- Seasonings of choice
- ½Avocado, slice

INSTRUCTIONS

1. Apply heat to oil in a big skillet over an average heat. Add mushrooms and fry for about 15 minutes. Remove the mushrooms from the pot and set aside.
2. Add butter to bread over medium high heat. Add the link to the bread for a total of about 5 minutes and brown all sides. If you

increase the size of the link, slice the center vertically and fry that way. The rinks are already cooked and enjoyable cold, but the sandwich is now fine.

3. While the links are brown, toast the English muffins and spread with your favorite seasoning such as Chipotle Mayo, which does not contain dairy products. Stack the fried mushrooms, rink and avocado with the english muffin slice top.

TO THE POWER OF OATS FOR FOUR NIGHTS

Active time: 10 minutes

Staying time: 8 hours

Total time: 8 hours 10 minutes

Yield: 2 YIELD

Protein: 23 grams per serving

If you've never eaten oats overnight, here's a great recipe to believe you. It is simple to the next order and uses the **INGREDIENTS** that everyone likes.

INGREDIENTS

- 3.5 cups of unsweetened almond milk
- 2 cups of traditional oats
- ¼ cup maple syrup
- 2 tablespoons of chia seeds
- 2 tablespoons unsweetened shredder coconut
- ¼ cup sunflower seed kernel
- 4 tablespoons peanut butter, split
- Sunflower seed kernel for garnish (optional)

INSTRUCTIONS

1. Add 2 tablespoons peanut butter and all ingredients except sunflower seeds to a large bowl. Mix well. It looks very wet, but chia seeds and oats absorb some of the milk. Cover and place in the refrigerator overnight.
2. Sprinkle two cups of peanut butter inside the two bowls to serve in the morning, each with oats overnight. Decorate with sunflower seeds if necessary.

RAW DATE CHOCOLATE BALLS

Active Time: 20 minutes
Refrigerator Time: 30 minutes
Total Time: 50 minutes
Yield: 24 balls

Protein: 6 grams per serving (2 balls)

These perfect little bites are made with the best variety of ingredients. They are sweet, crunchy, and chocolaty.

INGREDIENTS

- ¾ cup sunflower seed kernels, ground
- ½ cup dates, pitted, chopped well
- ½ cup walnuts, chopped
- ½ cup unsweetened cacao powder
- ½ cup maple syrup
- ½ cup creamy almond butter
- ½ cup old-fashioned oats (use gluten-free if desired)
- ¼ cup raw shelled hempseed

- 6 ounces unsweetened coconut, for coating

INSTRUCTIONS

1. Place the sunflower seeds, dates, walnuts, cacao powder, maple syrup, almond butter, oats, and hempseed in a large bowl. Mix well.
2. cut in pieces the dough and wrap into twenty-four balls. Roll each ball in shredded coconut. Place in the refrigerator to harden for about 30 minutes.

NO-BAKE CHOCOLATE PEANUT BUTTER COOKIES

Active Time: 5 minutes
Resting Time: 1 hour
Cook time: 5 minutes
Total Time: 1 hour 10 minutes
Yield: 24 cookies

Protein: 7 grams per serving (2 cookies)

Although these are no-bake cookies, they have the texture of baked cookies. They have no refined sugar, take 10 minutes to make, and are a favorite. That's a five-star rating!

INGREDIENTS

- ½ cup unsweetened dairy-free milk
- 3 tablespoons dairy-free butter
- ⅓ cup coconut sugar
- 1 tablespoon unsweetened cocoa powder
- ⅓ cup dairy-free semi-sweet chocolate chips
- 1 teaspoon vanilla extract
- ⅓ cup creamy peanut butter
- Pinch of salt
- 2½ cups old-fashioned oats or quick-cooking oats

- ¼ cup raw shelled hempseed

INSTRUCTIONS

1. Line a baking sheet with wax paper.
2. Place the milk, butter, sugar, cocoa powder, and chocolate chips in a large saucepan. Put on a rolling boil and time it. Let boil for 2 minutes. Stir occasionally so that the chocolate chips don't stick to the bottom of the pan before they melt. Remove from the heat and add the vanilla, peanut butter, and salt and mix until the peanut butter melts. Stir in the oats and hempseed.
3. Drop flour dollops onto the prepared baking sheet with one spoon. You will take them in a minute or less, and transform them into cookies. Let the cookies set for around an hour. Placing them in the refrigerator can accelerate the cooling and hardening process.

OVER-THE-TOP BARS TO GO

Active Time: 20 minutes
Refrigerator Time: 30 minutes
Cook time: 15 minutes
Total Time: 1 hour 5 minutes
Yield: 16 squares

Protein: 13 grams per serving (2 squares)

Not only are these bars gorgeous, but they travel really well, too. The ingredients are fun because they contain just about every nut and seed that you can think of.

INGREDIENTS

- 1½ cups old-fashioned oats
- ½ cup pecans
- ½ cup pistachios
- ½ cup cashews
- ½ cup dried cranberries
- ¼ cup dates, pitted and chopped
- ¼ cup sunflower seed kernels
- ¼ cup pepitas
- 2 tablespoons raw shelled hempseed
- ½ cup peanut butter
- ½ cup brown rice syrup
- 3 tablespoons maple syrup

INSTRUCTIONS

1. Cover square baking bowl with parchment paper and come up about 3 inches on opposite sides. This will act as a handle to remove the bars from the dish.
2. Mix all the ingredients except the peanut butter and the syrups together in a large bowl. Add the peanut butter and start to mix in with a wooden spoon, and then use your hands to mix and pinch so that the peanut butter is well incorporated into the dry ingredients.
3. Add the brown rice syrup and maple syrup to a small saucepan. Bring to a boil and cook to hard ball stage, 260°F, on a candy thermometer. Pour the syrups over the oat mixture and stir well. Then quickly spread the mixture into the prepared dish. It will cool quickly, so you can use your fingertips to press down into the dish as evenly as possible. You can also use the bottom of a measuring cup to press down firmly. Refrigerate for at least 30 minutes.
4. Grab the "handles" of the parchment paper and lift out of the

dish. Put on a cutting board and slice into16 squares.

PACKED PEANUT OATMEAL COOKIES

Active Time: 15 minutes
Cook time: 11 minutes
Total Time: 26 minutes
Yield: 12 YIELD

Protein: 8 grams per serving (2 cookies)

Peanuts, oats, and dairy-free cream are just the beginning of making a classic cookie that's packed with protein. What's more, they hardly take any time to make!

INGREDIENTS

- 1 tablespoon chia seeds or ground chia seeds
- 1 cups whole wheat flour
- 1 teaspoon baking powder
- 1½ cups old-fashioned oats
- 2 tablespoons vanilla protein powder
- ½ cup dairy-free butter
- 1 cup coconut sugar
- ½ cup dairy-free cream, softened
- 1 teaspoon vanilla extract
- 1 banana
- 1 cup peanuts, chopped

INSTRUCTIONS

1. Preheat the oven to 400°F. Cut parchment paper to fit on a baking sheet. Set aside.
2. Mix the chia seeds with 3 tablespoons water and set aside.

3. Add the flour, baking powder, oats, and protein powder to a large bowl. Set aside.
4. Mix the butter and sugar to the bowl of a stand mixer. Cream on medium-low speed for 5 minutes. Add the cream and mix well. Turn off the beater and add the prepared chia seed mixture, vanilla, and banana. Mix well on medium speed. Add the dry ingredients and peanuts and keep mixing until just combined.
5. Spoon dollops on a cookie sheet 2 inches apart and flatten with the bottom of a glass to about ½-inch thick. Bake for 11 minutes.
6. Cool on a wire rack.

HIGH-PROTEIN PEANUT BUTTER COOKIE DOUGH

Active Time: 15 minutes
Total Time: 15 minutes
Yield: 45 balls

Protein: 6¾ grams per serving (2 balls)

Here's a simple and delicious recipe. With a few ingredients and about 15 minutes you can satisfy your sweet tooth.

INGREDIENTS

- 1 cup crunchy peanut butter
- 1 cup maple syrup
- ½ teaspoon salt
- 1 cup chickpea flour
- ¾ cup almond meal flour
- ½ cup peanuts, chopped
- ½ cup cashews, chopped
- ½ cup old-fashioned oats
- Finely ground peanuts, for coating (optional)

INSTRUCTIONS

1. Mix the peanut butter and the syrup in a large bowl. Add the remaining ingredients and mix well. Shape into balls and eat.
2. If you'd like a little bit more of a refined look for serving, roll the balls into finely ground peanuts. For easier handling, store in the refrigerator between snacking.

BROCCOLI STIR-FRY WITH SEITAN AND CASHEWS

Active Time: 10 minutes
Cook time: 20 minutes
Total Time: 30 minutes
Yield: 2 YIELD

Protein: 43 grams per serving

A sweet and tangy sauce combined with veggies and cashews makes this an impressive dish. Serve over sticky jasmine rice for the perfect finish.

INGREDIENTS

- 1 cup jasmine rice
- 2 cups broccoli, stems peeled and diced, florets cut into bite-size pieces
- ½ cup tamari
- 2 tablespoons rice vinegar
- 2 tablespoons maple syrup
- ½ teaspoon ground ginger
- ¼ teaspoon garlic powder
- 1 red bell pepper, diced
- 2 tablespoons cornstarch or potato starch

- ¾ cup Pressure Cooker Thai Nuggets
- ½ cup raw cashews

INSTRUCTIONS

1. Add the rice and transfer 2 cups of water to a medium pot. Boil and cover while minimizing the heat and cook for about 20 minutes or until water is absorbed and the rice is soft.
2. In the meantime, add water to a medium-sized pot using a steamer and boil. Add the broccoli to the fill and steam with boiling water for 5 minutes. Remove from steamer and set aside.
3. In a small bowl, mix together the tamari, ¼ cup plus 2 tablespoons water, vinegar, syrup, ginger, and garlic powder.
4. Add 1 tablespoon sauce mixture to a large skillet. Turn the heat up to medium high and add bell peppers. Sauté for 5 minutes. Add the broccoli and cook for 5 minutes. Push the vegetables to the side and add cornstarch to the liquid. Leaving on medium-high heat, stir for 1 minute. Mix all together and add seitan nuggets and cashews. Cook to heat through for about 3 minutes.
5. Serve over the jasmine rice.

PROTEIN POWER GRILLED VEGGIE AND FRUIT SKEWERS

Active Time: 15 minutes
Cook time: 25 minutes
Total Time: 40 minutes
Yield: 4 YIELD

Protein: 16 grams per serving (2 skewers)

We all heard of fruit skewers, but have you heard of fruit and marinated tofu skewers? Everything is grilled on sticks to make the best fresh finger food.

INGREDIENTS

- 8 oz hard tofu, drainer, pressed, cut into 1-inch cubes
- 1 tablespoon vinegar
- 1 tablespoon of maple syrup
- 1/4 teaspoon chili powder
- 1 large sweet potato, peeled and chopped into bite-sized chunks
- 4 oz cremini mushroom
- 1 pineapple, chopped into chunks
- 1 red bell pepper, large chopped
- 1 yellow pepper, large chopped
- Extra virgin olive oil for grilling

INSTRUCTIONS

1. Place the cubes of tofu into a large bowl. Combine the tamari, rice vinegar, maple syrup, and chili powder together in a small bowl, and spill over tofu. 30 Minutes to Marinate.
2. Parboil the blocks of sweet potato for 10 minutes, or until tender.
3. Clean the mushrooms, and cut off the stem ends. Cut into halves or thirds, if some of the mushrooms are huge.
2. Skewer the tofu onto each skewer, sweet potato, pineapple, red and yellow bell peppers, and mushrooms.
5. Brush the grill with oil or grill pan and put to medium and high heat. Grill the skewered fruits and vegetables until the grill marks are visible. Flip the other side, and grill it.

CHICKPEA SALAD CROSTINI

Active Time: 15 minutes
Cook time: 5 minutes
Total Time: 20 minutes
Yield: 6 YIELD

Protein: 8½ grams per serving (2 crostini)

This appetizer ends with fresh, toasted slices of Italian bread. Finish that off with sweet marinated vegetables marinated with citrus and you have a good finger food.

INGREDIENTS

- 1 baguette, cut into 12 slices
- 2 tablespoons of extra virgin olive oil
- 115-ounce of chickpeas, drained and rinsed
- 115-ounce of black beans, drained and rinsed
- 18-ounce of corn, drained and rinsed 14-ounce of black olives, drained and sliced
- 1 tablespoon of fresh lime juice
- 2 tablespoons of flaxseed meal
- 1 teaspoon of ground cumin
- 1/4 teaspoon of chili powder
- 1/4 teaspoon of onion powder
- 1/4 teaspoon salt

INSTRUCTIONS

1. Lay the slices of bread out on a baking sheet. Brush every slice of bread with oil, lightly. (The new silicone brushes are perfect for this and they're really easy to wash up.) Put the baking sheet under the broiler. Don't do the rest. Just stand there and start to test the bread, and don't let it burn. It only requires a few minutes. Take off the sheet from the oven after the toasts are lightly browned. You can make these in advance, and also keep them in the fridge for later use.

To Construct

2. Mix all remaining ingredients together in a large bowl, except for the thyme.

3. Just before serving, top each toast with chickpea mixture. Add fresh thyme to garnish.

THAI SWEET CHILI TOFU STACKS

Active Time: 30 minutes
Cook time: 15 minutes
Total Time: 45 minutes
Yield: 6 YIELD

Protein: 9 grams per serving (4 stacks)

Make your life easier by using some of the prepackaged ingredients in preparation for a gathering. You and your guests will enjoy these stunning marinated tofu skewers, with plenty of flavor in every slice.

INGREDIENTS

- 1 tablespoon of cornstarch
- 1/2 cup of rice vinegar
- 1/2 cup of coconut sugar
- 1 chili pepper, such as jalapeño or cayenne, chopped fine
- 2 cloves of garlic, chopped fine
- 2 teaspoons of tamari
- 1/2 teaspoon of chopped parsley
- 1/4 teaspoon of cayenne pepper
- 8 ounces of extra firm tofu, washed, pressed and sliced into 1 inch cubes
- 18-ounce of pineapple

INSTRUCTIONS

1. Mix the cornstarch and 1 tablespoon of water together until smooth and set aside to prepare the sauce.
2. To a food processor, add the rice vinegar, 2/3 cup water, sugar, chili pepper, garlic, tamari, parsley, and cayenne pepper. Cook until the chili pepper is well mixed and very well broken up.
3. Pour the mixture into a small saucepan and heat until it boils, stirring until it dissolves the sugar. Turn heat off, and simmer for 5 minutes. Attach the cornstarch mixture and periodically stir for about 5 minutes or until the mixture has thickened a little. Remove

heat, and let it cool.
4. Remove the tofu cubes to the chili sauce, which is cooled. Let marinate for approximately 30 minutes.
5. Drain the pineapple and slice the rings into wedges of around 1- to 11/4 inches.
6. Place a slice of pineapple on a plate and center on top with a cube of marinated tofu. Place another slice of pineapple on the tofu, and with a toothpick safe.

SPICY CHICKPEA SEITAN TOFU ROLLUPS

Active Time: 20 minutes
Cook time: 5 minutes
Total Time: 25 minutes
Yield: 6 YIELD

Protein: 11 grams per serving (2 rollups)

For those protein-rich rollups, a super simple process and easy handling are two pluses. Tofu mixes with delicious ingredients to form a great base.

INGREDIENTS

- 2 ounces extra firm tofu, drained and pressed
- 1 cup canned chickpeas, drained and rinsed
- 2 tablespoons of dairy-free chipotle mayonnaise
- 1 tablespoon hot sauce
- 2 teaspoons hempseed, toasted in shell
- 2 teaspoons tahini
- 1/2 teaspoon cider vinegar
- 1/2 teaspoon garlic powder
- 1 green onion, chopped
- 1/4 teaspoon salt Pinch of ground black pepper
- 1/2 cup Steamed Seitan Smoky Nuggets
- 2 big spinach

INSTRUCTIONS

1. In a food processor add the tofu, chickpeas, mayonnaise, hot sauce, hempseed, tahini, vinegar, garlic powder, onion, salt and pepper. Cook with a knife until well combined and spreadable.
2. Chop in very small pieces of seitan nuggets. (You might also pulse a few times in a food processor.) Fry seitan in a small skillet over medium - high heat for about 4 minutes, stirring frequently to prevent burning. Deposit aside.
3. Divide the tofu filling into two pieces and evenly spread over each tortilla. Leave on one side about an inch off the edge without filling to assist in rolling. Sprinkle with seitan over every tortilla. Start rolling each tortilla to the opposite side of the edge you haven't covered. Roll firmly but not too tight, so that the filling does not squeeze out.
4. Place toothpicks about 11/2 to 2 inches apart along the bottom of the tortilla. Slice every toothpick between. This helps keep the rolls together until you are able to put them on a platter. They do stick very well together. When needed, garnish with fresh parsley.

CUCUMBER SEITAN ROLLUPS

Active Time: 15 minutes
Cook time: 15 minutes
Total Time: 30 minutes
Yield: 6 YIELD

Protein: 6 grams per serving (2 rollups)

Everyone will want to pick up one of those pretty little rolls of protein and veggies. Pop one in your mouth and enjoy the texture and flavours.

INGREDIENTS

- 1 red bell pepper
- 1 orange pepper
- 1 yellow bell pepper

- 26-inch cucumbers
- 1/4 cup hummus
- 1/4 teaspoon salt
- 1/4 teaspoon black pepper
- 1/3 cup seitan, crumbled

INSTRUCTIONS

1. Slice the bell peppers until each color has eighteen thin toothpick strips, then chop the remaining peppers into a very fine dice (there should be at least 3 tablespoons of each color; you might have some leftover). Deposit back.
2. Use a vegetable peeler to slice out the cucumbers with long stripes. Hold the same direction so that every long edge of the strips will have some colour. Slice on all four sides and cut seed segment in the middle. Of each of the cucumber's four sides, you will have about two or three slices.
3. Lay those slices out. Place about 2 teaspoons of hummus down the center of each strip; place out thinly, holding off the long edge a little. Sprinkle a dash of salt and pepper on each cucumber that is covered with hummus. Now scatter on each slice about 11/2 teaspoons of seitan and sliced bell pepper blend.
4. Roll each cucumber up with a toothpick and secure it. Set on their sides and at various heights slide three separate-colored bell pepper strips into the centre. To achieve that look, you'll need to cut some of them shorter.

LENTIL BALLS IN SWEET AND SPICY RED SAUCE

Active Time: 20 minutes
Cook time: 45 minutes
Total Time: 1 hour 5 minutes
Yield: 6 YIELD

Protein: 12 grams per serving (3 lentil balls)

For this appetizer a crispy lentil bean ball rolls mixed in a tangy tomato sauce. Make sure you've got napkins and toothpicks on hand so you won't need a leftover bottle.

INGREDIENTS

Lentil Balls

- 3/4 cup green lentils
- 11/2 cups vegetable broth
- 2 teaspoons of extra virgin olive oil
- 1/3 cup diced onion
- 1/3 cup fast-cooking oats
- 2 cups of grated carrots
- 2 cloves of garlic, finely chopped
- 2 tablespoons of tomato paste
- 1 tablespoon aquafaba
- 3/4 teaspoon Italian seasoning
- 3/4 teaspoon salt
- Pinch of ground black pepper
- Sweet and Spicy Sauce
- 1/4 cup diced onion
- 1 15-ounce fire-roasted tomatoes

INSTRUCTIONS

1. Rinse lentils, and drain them. Place the lentils in a medium-large casserole. Pour in and cover with vegetable broth. Place the saucepan over high heat and bring to a boil. Turn to medium height when cooking, and simmer for 20 minutes or until the lentils are tender. They should absorb all of the water. This can be done in a rice cooker, too.
2. Preheat to 425 ° F on burner.
3. Heat up the oil over medium to high heat in a small skillet. Stir in the onion and sauté, about 10 to 15 minutes, until translucent.
4. In a large bowl, add the cooked lentils, sautéed onions, peas, carrots, garlic, tomato paste, aquafaba, Italian seasoning, salt, and pepper. Mix and mix well.

5. Form lentil mixture parts into eighteen balls, and put them on a baking sheet. Bake for 10 minutes, flip, then bake for another 10 minutes.
Sweet and pungent Sauce 6. Add all the ingredients in the sauce to a food processor. Mix well until smooth. Small pieces of pineapple still should be present.
7. Pour over into a large casserole. Switch to medium heat and carry to a boil.
8. Carefully fill the pan with lentil balls and fold them into the sauce. Heat up for about five minutes, then serve with toothpicks.

CHICKPEA BALL POPPERS

Active Time: 15 minutes
Cook time: 25 minutes
Total Time: 40 minutes
Yield: 6 YIELD

Protein: 10 grams per serving (4 ball poppers)

Those little balls have so many delicious flavors wrapped up. Not just that! A sweet vegan mayo dip is also available to go right alongside.

INGREDIENTS

- Chickpea Balls
- 1 28-ounce can be chickpeas, drained (save the liquid to be used as aquafaba) and rinsed
- 1 teaspoon tamari
- 2 teaspoons onion powder
- 1 teaspoon salt
- 1/2 teaspoon ground black pepper
- 4 tablespoons aquafaba
- 1 cup of fresh breadcrumbs Spicy Mayo Dip
- 1/2 cup vegan mayonnaise

- 1/4 cup sweet chili sauce
- 1 teaspoon tamari
- 1/2 teaspoon Tabasco

INSTRUCTIONS

1. Preheat to 400 ° F on oven.
2. Add all the ingredients in the chickpea ball to a food processor. Pulse until the chickpeas break down and the ingredients blend. Form mixture into 24 bean balls and place on a baking sheet. Bake for another 25 minutes.
Spicy Dip mayo 3. Thoroughly mix all the ingredients for dip.
4. Serve alongside chickpea ball poppers in a bowl of toothpicks.

ENGLISH MUFFIN PROTEIN TRIANGLES

Soaking Time: 1 hour
Active Time: 20 minutes
Cook time: 2 minutes
Total Time: 1 hour 20 minutes
Yield: 6 YIELD

Protein: 12 grams per serving (4 triangles)

Here's a special, simple to make appetizer. Flavor-packed flavors are piled high on English muffins and mixed together. You have bite-size treats after broiling and slicing which you will want to serve over and over again.

INGREDIENTS

- 3 English muffins
- 2/3 cup raw almonds, soaked in water from one hour to one overnight
- 11/2 tablespoons lemon juice
- 11/2 tablespoons nutritional leaves 1 teaspoon curry powder

- 1/2 teaspoon mustard powder
- 1/2 teaspoon salt Pinch of ground black pepper
- 1/3 cup extra virgin olive oil, more if desired
- 1/3 cup seitan, crumbled
- 1/4 cup black olives, sliced
- Freshly cut parsley, for garnish (optional)

INSTRUCTIONS

1. In the middle break away the English muffins and toast. Place and set aside on baking sheet.
2. Insert the almonds into a food processor. Remove the juice of lemon, nutritious leaven, curry paste, mustard powder, salt and pepper. Blend as smooth as you can until the mixture gets. It still has a couple of small bits. Little by little, pour in the olive oil through the lid opening. If you want it thinner you can add a little more oil. Pour the mixture into a small bowl, then add the crumbled seitan together.
3. Divide the paste, scattered over the six halves of muffins. It is going to be very dense. Slide the baking sheet under the broiler for about 2 minutes, until white.
4. Top with slices of black olive, and cut into quarters each muffin. The easiest way to do this is to use a cleaver and push straight as you'd cut pizza. Place on a tray, and garnish, if desired, with freshly cut parsley.

HEARTS FLAXSEED ON PEACH YOGURT

Active Time: 10 minutes
Cook Time: 5 minutes
Total Time: 15 minutes
YIELD: 1

Protein: 10 grams per serving

INGREDIENTS

- Flaxseed
- 1 heart shaped cutter
- Peach jam
- Assorted Nuts
- 1 200cc peach yogurt

INSTRUCTIONS

1. Cut it in a heart shape, reserve.
2. In a bowl, place the pudding hearts; add a teaspoon of jam to each Almonds and blueberries
3. Add the peach yogurt very cold to the source without touching the hearts, in the background
4. Enjoy this delicious snack

ALMOND AND BRUSSELS SPROUTS

Active Time: 15 minutes
Cook Time: 10 minutes
Total Time: 25 minutes
YIELD: **4**

Protein: 12 grams per serving

INGREDIENTS

- Brussels sprouts 700 g
- 100 g chopped almonds
- 1 large garlic piece-half
- Untreated lemon 1 zest-minced
- Organic margarine 50 g
- 2 tablespoons of bread crumbs

- Salt and pepper

INSTRUCTIONS

1. Clean the Brussels sprouts, cut off the bottom edge and cut it diagonally. Add boiling salt water and cook for 5-7 minutes. Drain the cooking water and cover the cabbage.
2. Heat half of the margarine in a frying pan, add almonds and garlic, and roast for about 3 minutes. Next, add lemon peel, salt and pepper. Remove half of the garlic and remove the pan from the fire.
3. Heat the remaining margarine in a small pan, toast the bread crumbs in golden color and add to the almond mixture.
4. Distribute and serve everything on Brussels sprouts.

POTATOES WITH ZUCCHINI, EGGPLANT AND HERBS

Active Time: 10 minutes
Cook Time: 20 minutes
Total Time: 30 minutes
YIELD: **3**

Protein: 8 grams per serving (2 cookies)

INGREDIENTS

- Potatoes about 600 - 700 g
- 1 zucchini
- 1 eggplant
- 1 - 2 toes of fresh garlic
- 150 ml of coconut milk
- 2 - 3 tablespoons rapeseed oil
- 10 - 15 salted macadamia nuts
- 5 - 10 small branches of thyme
- 5 small branches of rosemary
- 1/2 teaspoon ginger ground

- 1/2 teaspoon curry powder
- 1/2 teaspoon turmeric ground
- Salt pepper

INSTRUCTIONS

1. Cut the potatoes, zucchini and aubergine into small pieces. Then cut the vegetables into small cubes to make it faster, and we also find it more appetizing.
2. Put everything together in a bowl and squeeze garlic.
3. Everything is blended well with the oil, spices, salt and pepper.
4. Then prepare the whole thing early so that the spices can move in well.
5. Then spread in the Omnia, put the herb branches in between, the macadamia nuts chopped over sprinkle with salt and pepper seasoning on top.
6. At 20 min at the highest level, potato is ready, serve.

SPINACH AND FETA FRITTATA

Active Time: 15 minutes
Cook Time: 15 minutes
Total Time: 30 minutes
Serving: 2

Protein: 18 grams per serving

INGREDIENTS

- 1 potato, peel and cut large
- 6 eggs
- Olive oil
- 1 small chopped shallot

- 10-12 grape tomatoes cut in half
- Handful of spinach
- ¼ cup feta
- Salt and pepper

INSTRUCTIONS

1. Preheat the oven to 350 degrees.
2. Put the potato pieces in a pan and cover with 1-2 inches of cold water. Heat to medium high heat and bring to a boil. As soon as the water boils, turn off the power and drain the potatoes.
3. In the meantime, mix the eggs well in a bowl so that they shine slightly.

Season with salt and pepper

4. Heat a large pot (10 inches) for the oven and cover the bottom with olive oil. Stir the potatoes until they are golden and stir frequently for about 5 minutes.
5. Season with salt and pepper and add shallots. Cut into cubes, soften slightly towards the end, and brown.
6. If necessary, add olive oil before pouring eggs into frying potatoes and shallots. 7. Spread the spinach, tomatoes and feta evenly.

Cook the fritters on medium heat for a few minutes, then transfer to the oven and continue cooking for 6-10 minutes until the eggs are cooked but not brown.

8. Slide the tray on the plate and cut it into small pieces.

SKYR WITH KERNELS, GRAPEFRUIT AND KIWI

Active Time: 15 minutes
Cook time: 5 minutes
Total Time: 20 minutes
Yield: 4

Protein: 6 grams per serving

INGREDIENTS

- 15g pistachio nuts (1 tbsp)
- 15g almonds (1 tbsp)
- 15g walnut kernels (1 tbsp)
- 15g cashews (1 tbsp)
- 10g coconut chips (1 tbsp)
- 1grapefruit or blood orange
- 2 kiwis
- 800g skyr
- 8 g puffed amaranth (2 tbsp)

INSTRUCTIONS

1. Fry the cores and coconut chips in a hot pan over medium heat without fat for 3-4 minutes. Take out and put aside.

2. Slice the grapefruit, quarter the slices and peel as desired. Peel and slice the kiwis.

3. Fill skyr into 4 small bowls and add fruit, sprinkle with kernels and amaranth and serve.

CARROT PATTY

Active Time: 10 minutes
Cook Time: 10 minutes
Total Time: 20 minutes
YIELD: **2**

Protein: 8 grams per serving

INGREDIENTS

- 100 g carrots
- 50 g of potatoes
- 1 egg (size M)
- 5 g cornstarch
- salt
- pepper
- ¼ bunch of chives
- 2 tablespoons oil
- 50 g of zucchini
- 3 teaspoons olive oil
- 1 fry tomato (about 125 g)
- ½ organic lemon
- 50 g of sour cream
- 25 ml of milk
- 1 pinch of sugar
- 10 g rocket

INSTRUCTIONS

1. Grate carrots and potatoes roughly. Mix carrots, potatoes, egg and starch, season. Wash the chives, cut into small rolls and put them under the patties. Heat oil in a pan. Form the pancake and sauté from both sides for about 10 minutes.

2. Cut the zucchini into thin slices, season. Heat olive oil in a pan. Fry zucchini in it.

3. Slice tomato. Remove lemon zest, squeeze out. Mix sour cream with lemon zest, 1 teaspoon juice and milk. Season with sugar, salt and pepper. Serve patty with tomato, zucchini slices and rocket. Pour lemon sauce over it.

POTATO-HACK SOUP WITH MUSHROOMS

Active Time: 25 minutes
Cook Time: 15 minutes
Total Time: 40 minutes
YIELD: **4**

INGREDIENTS

- 600 g predominantly hard-boiling potatoes
- 200 g leek (1 small stick)
- 2 tbsp rapeseed oil
- 800 ml vegetable stock
- salt
- ½ tl ground caraway
- 200 g mushrooms
- ½ tl dried marjoram
- 200 g whipped cream
- 20 g parsley (0.5 bunch)
- 40 g walnuts

INSTRUCTIONS

1. Peel potatoes, wash and cut into small cubes. Clean leeks, wash, halve lengthways and cut into fine rings.
2. Heat 1 tbsp of rape seed oil in a saucepan, add the potatoes and the leek and fry for 3-4 minutes over medium heat. Pour with the broth, season with salt and cumin and cook for 10-15 minutes.
3. Meanwhile mushrooms clean, wash if necessary and cut into slices. Heat remaining oil in a pan, add the mushrooms and fry for another 3 minutes. Season with marjoram, salt and cumin.
4. Add the cream and the mushroom mince to the soup, stir and heat. Wash parsley, shake dry and chop. Roughly chop walnuts. Serve with garnished soup with parsley and walnuts.

CREAMY PUMPKIN SOUP WITH NUTS

Active Time: 30 minutes
Cook Time: 15 minutes
Total Time: 45 minutes
Yield: 4

Protein: 6 grams per serving
INGREDIENTS

- 150 g potatoes
- 400 g pumpkin pulp
- 1 onion
- 1 clove of garlic
- 2 tbsp butter
- 1 tsp curry powder
- 750 ml vegetable stock
- 3 tbsp pecans
- 200 g sour cream
- salt

- cayenne pepper
- nutmeg

INSTRUCTIONS

1. Peel and dice the potatoes. Also dice the pumpkin pulp. Peel the onion and garlic, finely chop, fry in hot butter, then add the squash cubes and curry and fry briefly.
2. Pour the stock, add the potatoes to the saucepan and simmer over low heat for 25-30 minutes.
3. Roast the pecans in a pan without fat until they smell sweet. Take out and chop small.

Puree the soup and, depending on the desired consistency, stir in broth or simmer. 4. Stir in 150 g of sour cream, puree again and do not cook. Season with salt, cayenne pepper and fresh grated nutmeg.

5. Fill the soup in bowls, stir in 1 tbsp of remaining sour cream and add B. with a stick in streaks pull. Serve with nuts sprinkled with nuts.

BALSAMIC ROASTED VEGETABLES

Active Time: 30 minutes
Cook Time: 20 minutes
Total Time: 50 minutes
YIELD: **4**

Protein: 6 grams per serving

INGREDIENTS

- 0.5dl Balsamic Vinegar
- 100g feta

- 50g eggplant
- 50g red onions
- 50g green pepper
- 50g red pepper
- A bit of salt
- Some rosemary

INSTRUCTIONS

1. Preheat the oven to 200ºC.
2. Cut the vegetables into irregular pieces.
3. Peel the potatoes and cut into thick slices.
4. Season with olive oil, salt, rosemary and vinegar
5. Put in the oven for 20 minutes.
6. Before serving, crumble the feta over the vegetables and drizzle with some Gallo Balsamic Vinegar.

TORTILLA AND PEAS

Active Time: 20 minutes
Cook Time: 20 minutes
Total Time: 40 minutes
YIELD: **4**

Protein: 10 grams per serving

INGREDIENTS

- 100 ml of milk
- Salt pepper
- 50 g mashed potatoes
- 150 g of frozen peas
- 1 bunch of parsley

- 8 eggs (size Medium)
- 2 shallots
- 2 tbsp olive oil

INSTRUCTIONS

1. Preheat oven (electric cooker: 200 ° C / circulating air: 175 ° C / gas: see manufacturer). Boil milk, 150 ml water and 1/4 teaspoon salt. Remove from heat, 2. stir in purée flakes. Brew frozen peas with boiling water, quench.

3. Wash parsley, chop. Whisk eggs and potato mixture, season. Add peas and parsley.

4. Peel the shallots, dice. Heat the oil in an oven-proof pan. Steam the shallots in it. 5. Add egg mass. Stir in the oven for about 15 minutes, serve.

COLOURFUL WRAPS WITH VEGETABLES

Active Time: 20 minutes
Cook Time: 10 minutes
Total Time: 30 minutes
YIELD: **4**

Protein: 6 grams per serving

INGREDIENTS

- 40 g baby spinach
- 1carrot
- 40 g cheddar (1 piece, 45% fat in dry matter)
- salt
- pepper
- 4 whole wheat tortilla

INSTRUCTIONS

1. Wash spinach and spin dry. Clean the carrot, peel and cut into thin slices with a peeler. Cheddar rubs.
2. Stir cream with salt and pepper. Spread tortillas with cheddar, spinach and carrot over the tortillas. Fold the two short sides of the tortilla onto the filling, then fold in the long side and roll to the open side to wraps.
3. Roast tortillas in a hot pan from both sides for 2-3 minutes to the desired degree of browning and serve immediately.

RATATOUILLE

Active Time: 50 minutes
Cooking time: 40 minutes
Total time: 90 minutes
Serving: 6

Protein: 8 grams per serving

INGREDIENTS

- 300 g zucchini (1 zucchini)
- 300 g eggplant (1 eggplant)
- salt
- 800 g pepper (2 red + 2 yellow 4 peppers)
- 2 stems basil
- 2 branches thyme
- 2 onions
- 2 garlic cloves
- 3 tbsp olive oil
- 425 g pizza tomato (can)
- pepper
- 40 g parmesan (1 piece)

- 3 tbsp wholemeal breadcrumbs

INSTRUCTIONS

1. Wash the zucchini and aubergine, rub dry and cut into 5 mm thick slices. Sprinkle the cut surfaces with a little salt and let the vegetable slices soak for 15 minutes.
2. In the meantime, quarter the peppers, core them and wash them.
3. Wash herbs, shake dry, put aside 1 thyme sprig for garnish. Peel leaves and chop finely.
4. Peel onions and garlic and finely chop. Heat 1 teaspoon of oil in a pan. Lightly brown the onions and garlic in medium heat for 2-4 minutes.
5. Add pizza tomato and herbs, bring to a boil, season with salt and pepper, and put aside.
6. Dab zucchini and aubergine slices dry. Mix with chili quarters and remaining oil in a bowl. Grate the Parmesan and mix with the breadcrumbs.
7. Heat a grill pan and grill the vegetable slices in it for 1 minute from each side.
8. If necessary, grease the baking dish. Add vegetables and tomato sauce alternately. Bake in preheated oven at 200 ° C (circulating air: 180 ° C, gas: stage 3) for a total of 25 minutes, after 15 minutes sprinkle over parmesan crumbs. Garnish ratatouille with thyme.

OMELETTE AND SUMMER VEGETABLES

Active Time: 10 minutes
Cook Time: 15 minutes

Total Time: 25 minutes
YIELD: 1

Protein: 6 grams per serving

INGREDIENTS

- 1/4 cup frozen whole grain corn, thawed
- 1/3 cup chopped zucchini
- 3 tablespoons chopped green onion
- 2 tablespoons water
- 1/4 tsp black pepper or 1 tablespoon
- 2 Large Egg Whites
- 1 Large Whole Egg
- 1 ounce Low Fat Cheddar

INSTRUCTIONS

1. Heat a small pan over medium high heat. Apply cooking spray to the pan. Add corn, zucchini and onions to the pan. Stir for 4 minutes or until vegetables are soft and firm.
2. Remove from fire. Heat a 10-inch frying pan over medium high heat. Mix water, pepper, egg white and eggs in a bowl and mix well with a whisk. Apply cooking
3. spray to the pan. Pour the egg mixture into the pan.
4. Cook until the edges are firm (about 2 minutes). Gently lift the edge of the omelette with a spatula and tilt the pan so that the uncooked egg mixture touches the pan.
5. Using a spoon, place the vegetable mixture in half of the omelette and sprinkle the vegetables on the low fat cheddar mixture.
6. Remove the omelette with a spatula and fold the omelette in half. Bake for another 2 minutes or until the cheddar melts. Gently slide the omelette onto the plate.

BEAN PASTE
Active Time: 20 minutes
Cook Time: 40 minutes
Total Time: 1 hour
YIELD: **4**

Protein: 14 grams per serving

INGREDIENTS

- Lemon Juice
- Onion 1 Unit
- Paprika 20 g
- Black beans 100 g
- Salt Amount needed
- Garlic
- Parsley 10 g
- olive oil

INSTRUCTIONS

1. Soak black beans overnight in cold water with a chopped onion and a clove of garlic. Boil , strain and let cool.
2. Process the beans with salt, pepper, juice of lemon and olive oil. Garnish with parsley. Serve with toast.

WHITE BEAN DIP

Active Time: 15 minutes
Cook Time: 20 minutes
Total Time: 35 minutes
YIELD: 10

Protein: 16 grams per serving

INGREDIENTS

- 1 can (15 oz) beans drained
- 4 ounces (1/2 pack of 8 oz) Cream, softened
- 1/2 cup of Sour Cream
- 2 tablespoons chopped green chilli peppers
- 1 package (8 oz) of four-shredded Mexican style fine
- 3 green onions, chopped well

INSTRUCTIONS

1. Heat the oven to 350 ° F.
2. Grind the beans in a large bowl. Add cream, sour cream and chili peppers; mix well. Now add a cup of the to mix with the bean. Spread it in an 8-inch casserole dish or a refractory mold sprayed with oil spray.
3. Bake the dip 20 min. Sprinkle with the remaining; bake 5 min. more or until the melts.
4. Sprinkle with green onions. Serve the dip with the Crackers and an assortment of chopped vegetables.

RICE WITH BLACK BEANS AND PINEAPPLE

Active Time: 25 minutes
Cook Time: 15 minutes
Total Time: 40 minutes
YIELD: 6

Protein: 14 grams per serving

INGREDIENTS

- 3 cups chicken broth

- 1 cup long-grain white rice, washed uncooked and drained
- 1 can (15 oz) black beans, drained
- 1 cup chopped fresh pineapple
- 2 tablespoons grated Parmesan
- 1/4 cup fresh parsley, chopped

INSTRUCTIONS

1. Cook the red Stir Fry in a large pot for 3 min, intermittently turning it. Add the broth and rice; Let it boil. Cover the pot; Cook it, keeping a soft boil, over medium-low heat for 15 min.
2. Put the beans and pineapple on top. (Do not stir.) Cover the pot, cook them, keeping a soft boil, for 5 min. or until the rice is soft and the mixture is completely hot. Stir gently.
3. Sprinkle the dish with the parmesan and parsley.

CRISPY BAKED PUFFED TOFU WITH TERIYAKI SAUCE

Active Time: 10 minutes
Marinating Time: 1 hour
Cook time: 40 minutes
Total Time: 1 hour 50 minutes

Protein: 8 grams per serving (4 pieces)

Puffed tofu is a nice way to treat yourself to tofu. The result is crispy on the outside, seasoned and baked, and creamy on the inside.

INGREDIENTS

Puffed Tofu

- 7 ounces extra firm tofu, drained and pressed
- 1/2 cup vegetable broth
- 2 table spoons hot sauce
- 1/4 cup cornstarch Dipping Sauce
- 2 table spoons tamari

- 2 table spoons cornstarch
- 2 table spoons maple syrup
- 1/4 teaspoon garlic powder
- 1/4 teaspoon ground ginger

INSTRUCTIONS

Puffed Tofu

1. Flip the tofu on its side, and cut two rectangles through the middle. Flip them in and stack onto their smooth sides. Cut through the center, and cut those two halves twice each without separating the halves. Make two cuts lengthwise equal in size. There are now 24 cubes. Place the cubes in a small flat casserole platter or other container that will suit all the cubes on one surface.
2. Blend the vegetable broth and hot sauce together. Glue the tofu on. Marinate for about an hour.
3. Preheat to 350 ° F on oven.
4. In a medium bowl, placed 1/4 cup cornstarch. Cut the tofu and put on the cornstarch. Put the tofu on a baking sheet then toss. Bake 30-40 minutes. Toss every 10 minutes with a spatula, before golden and puffed.

Sauce Dip 5. Add 1/2 cup water, tamari, and cornstarch and medium - high heat to a small saucepan. Remove until cornstarch dissolves. Remove left ingredients and bring to a boil. Turn heat down to medium, and cook, stirring to desired thickness. Place the tofu on a toothpick platter and sprinkle with the sauce.

TRIPLE POWER PATTIES

Active Time: 25 minutes
Cook time: 55 minutes
Total Time: 1 hour 20 minutes
Yield: 6 YIELD

Protein: 6½ grams per serving (2 patties)

These patties are filled with so many delicious ingredients-but there's more! There's a spicy mayo dip for vegan too.

INGREDIENTS

Patties

- 2 small sweet potatoes, peeled and sliced in2-inch cubes (equal to 2 cups mashed sweet potato)
- 1 cup quinoa
- 2 table spoons extra virgin olive oil
- split 1/4 cup diced onion
- 2 table spoons raw shelled hempseed
- 1/4 teaspoon paprika
- 1/4 teaspoon ground cumin
- 1/4 cup panko
- 1 14-ounce can black beans, washed and rinsed
- 1/2 cup vegan mayonnaise
- 1/4 cup sweet chili sauce

INSTRUCTIONS

1. In a medium saucepan, place the sweet potato cubes, and cover with water. Cover and bring to a boil then turn down the heat to medium height. Cook a little smashed with the foil, around 15 minutes or until you are able to pierce the sweet potatoes with a fork. Mash and drain. Deposit aside.
2. Cook the quinoa in a different saucepan: put the quinoa in a sieve and rinse well. Combine the quinoa and 2/3 cup water in a small saucepan. Bring to a boil, cover and diminish to a simmer. Cook for 10 to 15 minutes, or until it absorbs the water. Remove from heat and allow to set for 5 minutes with the cover. Cut fluff and cover.
3. In the meantime, apply 1 tablespoon of oil to a pan, and heat up to hot. Add the onion and sauté, or until transparent, for about 10 to 15 minutes.
4. Add the mashed potatoes, quinoa, salted onion, hempseed, paprika, cumin and panko to a large bowl, and mix well. Stir in the

black beans Make twelve balls and then flatten to the about 1/4 inch thick patties.

5. Attach a pan with the remaining oil and fire to medium heat. Black the patties on each hand for about 3 to 5 minutes or until light brown.

Spicy Dip May 6. Thoroughly mix all the ingredients for dip.

7. Serve alongside Triple Power Patties in a bowl.

BLACK BEAN TEMPEH NACHOS WITH CASHEW

Active Time: 20 minutes
Soaking Time: 1 hour
Cook time: 10 minutes
Total Time: 1 hour 30 minutes
Yield: 4 YIELD

Protein: 27 grams per serving

This fabulous array of ingredients is more of a recipe than an assembly. The cashew is so delicious that by the spoonful you will want to eat it.

INGREDIENTS

Cashew

- 3/4 cup raw cashews, soaked from 1 hour to overnight and drained
- 1 table cup nutritional yeast
- 1 table cup tapioca starch or tapioca flour (they are the same thing)
- 1/2 teaspoon garlic powder
- 1/2 teaspoon onion powder
- 1 table cup lemon juice
- 1/2 cup water Tempeh Nachos

- 10 to 18 ounces tortilla chips
- 1 15-ounce black beans, drained and rinsed
- 1/2 cup red onion

INSTRUCTIONS

1. Apply all the ingredients in the to a blender and combine until creamy. Transfer this mixture blended into a small saucepan. Cook over medium heat and stir until the sauce gets a bit thick. It'll take 5 to 10 minutes to complete. Take the heat off to cool down somewhat.

To have Nachos

2 made. Place the chips on a plate. Sprinkle the chips over the black beans. Dot with cashew . Sprinkle all over the top of red onion, cabbage, tempeh, chili pepper and hemps.

3. Dice the avocado in lime juice, then dredge. Sprinkle over the nachos with diced avocado.

TOASTED PROTEIN MUSHROOM ROLLS

Active Time: 20 minutes
Soaking Time: 1 hour
Cook time: 15 minutes
Total Time: 1 hour 35 minutes
Yield: 6 YIELD

Protein: 18 grams per serving (3 rolls)

Here's one thing you've probably never seen before. Roll some flat bread, spread over filling, roll up, and bake. Whoa!

INGREDIENTS:

- ¼ cup raw cashews, soaked for 1 hour
- 1 tablespoon plus

- 2 teaspoons dairy-free milk
- 1 teaspoon lemon juice
- ¼ teaspoon salt Pinch of ground black pepper
- 4 ounces button mushrooms
- ¼ cup dairy-free oil, split
- 2 tablespoons raw shelled hempseed
- 9 slices whole-grain bread

INSTRUCTIONS

1. Add cashews, sugar, lemon juice, salt, and pepper to a food processor. Continue until smooth.
2. Clean the mushrooms, and chop them finely.
3. In a shallow skillet heat up 1 tablespoon butter over medium - high heat. Add chopped mushrooms and sauté for 5 minutes. Turn off the heat, then add the mixture of cashew and hempseed. Shake well.
4. Preheat to 425 ° F on oven.
5. Take crusts off of the bread and leave in a square shape. With a rolling pin roll every square thin. You are going to roll the squares around. Spread 1 spoonful of mushroom mixture over each square and roll up.
6. Melt remaining butter.
7. Cut rolls in half and roll in melted butter. Place the rolls on the cookie sheets and bake until browned for 8 minutes.

ARTICHOKE QUINOA DIP

Active Time: 20 minutes
Cook time: 25 minutes
Total Time: 45 minutes
Yield: 4 YIELD

Protein: 10 grams per serving

This is a fairly quick dive. It can also be used as a mini toast spread or stuffed into a variety of vegetables, such as mini bell peppers. All are good self-righteous appetizers.

INGREDIENTS

- 1/2 cup quinoa
- 1 tablespoon of extra virgin olive oil
- 1/2 cup of onion
- 4 ounces of baby spinach
- 1/4 cup of fresh shelled hempseed
- 1/2 teaspoon of onion powder
- 1/2 teaspoon of garlic powder
- 1 teaspoon of salt
- 1/4 teaspoon of ground black pepper
- 8 ounces of artichoke heart in broth
- 1 tablespoon of lemon juice

INSTRUCTIONS

1. Place the quinoa and rinse well in a sieve. In a small saucepan, add the quinoa and 1 cup of water. Bring to a boil, cover and reduce to a simmer. Cook for 10 to 15 minutes, or until it consumes the oil, Remove from heat and require to set for 5 minutes with the cover. Remove fluff and lid.
2. Steam up the oil over medium to high heat in a large skillet. Add the onion and sauté for 10 minutes, over medium heat. Stir in the spinach and simmer for about a minute or so, until wilted. Add the hempseed and spices, and quickly stir in. Out of heat remove.
3. Split off the heads of artichoke tops. Discard the outer leaves hardest.
4. Add all to food processor. System is very low until well mixed and sliced.
5. Serve with pita chips made homely (see note).

Note: Homemade pita chips are a very simple process: Buy a pita pocket bag or flatbread bag. Put oil in the pita pockets, and cut into triangles. Lay it down on a baking sheet. Bake for about 5-7 minutes at 400 ° F. Watch closely to ensure they are not burning.

VEGETABLE CREAM WITH CROUTONS

Active Time: 40 minutes
Cook Time: 35 minutes
Total Time: 1 hour 15 minutes
YIELD: **4**

Protein: 10 grams per serving

INGREDIENTS

- 70g onions
- 2 tbsp olive oil
- 150 ml of white wine
- 400 ml vegetable stock
- 250 ml whipped cream
- 100 g of Italian hard parmesan (eg Grana Padano , finely grated)
- Salt pepper
- nutmeg
- 2 tsp cornstarch
- 300 g box white bread, (from the previous day)
- 50 g butter
- 300 g of small firm potatoes
- 300 g of carrots
- 0.5 cauliflower, (about 400 g)
- 1 small broccoli, (about 350 g)
- 1 yellow zucchini, (about 200 g)
- 300 g peas, (alternatively 100 g frozen peas)
- 1 bunch chervil

INSTRUCTIONS

1. Finely chop the onions and fry in hot oil. Deglaze with white

wine and reduce to half. Fill with vegetable stock and cream and cook over medium heat for 5 minutes.
2. Add the parmesan and cook for a further 5 minutes with occasional stirring until the parmesan has melted. Mix finely with the cutting stick and season with salt, pepper and nutmeg. Mix the corn flour with 5 tablespoons of cold water and tie the sauce with it. Keep the sauce covered.
3. Slice the white bread into 2 cm slices, decortelize and cut into 2 cm cubes. Heat the butter in a large frying pan and roast the bread cubes in a medium heat while turning pale brown. Season the croutons with a bit of nutmeg and salt and immediately pour into a bowl.

4. Peel and halve the potatoes. Peel carrots and cut diagonally into 3-4 cm long pieces. Clean cauliflower and broccoli, cut florets from the stems. Clean the zucchini, cut them lengthwise and cut crosswise into pieces about 5 mm thick. Peas from pods
5. Boil potatoes in boiling salted water for 10-15 minutes, drain and steam. Cook carrots in 2 liters of lightly salted water over medium heat for 8 minutes. Add cauliflower and broccoli after 3 minutes.
6. Drain cooked vegetables in a well-drenched well. Bring the sauce to a boil and add the cooked vegetables, zucchini and peas and cook for another 3 minutes over a low heat. Then add the potatoes and leave everything for 3 minutes with the stove off. Pick up the chervil leaves.
7. Arrange vegetable ragout in a preheated bowl. Garnish with chervil leaves and serve immediately with the Muskatcroûtons.

BAKED SEITAN SWIRLS

Active Time: 15 minutes
Cook time: 15 minutes
Total Time: 30 minutes
Yield: 6 YIELD

Protein: 16 grams per serving (4 swirls)

These tender, robust bites are perfect for dipping. They are satisfying, rolled in with spicy seitan. Serve those swirls with your variety of sauces. You keep the heat under control.

INGREDIENTS:

- 1/2 cup of all-purpose flour
- 1/2 cup of whole wheat flour
- 1 tablespoon of coconut sugar
- 1 teaspoon of baking soda
- 1/4 teaspoon of salt
- 5 tablespoons of coconut oil, melted
- 6 tablespoons of dairy-free milk
- 8 ounces seitan (Slow Cooker Log for Thin Slices and Crumbles) Mustards, to be served:

INSTRUCTIONS

1. Preheat to 350 ° F on burner.
2. In a medium bowl, add the flours, sugar, baking powder, baking soda and salt. Blend well.
3. Combine the oil and milk in a small saucepan. Stir in the dry mixture to make the dough rigid.
4. Roll the dough out into a rectangle of about 8 inches. Cut the center lengthwise, so that two rectangles measuring 4 by 8 inches are present.
4. Put the seitan in a food processor and crumble for processing. Divide the seitan into half and spread over each rectangle of dough leaving 1 inch on each rectangle's long side. Start to roll up, lengthwise, and end at the edge where there is no seitan. Roll strong, but not stiffly. Cut hand seam. Split each roll into rolls of about 3/4 inches. You'll end up with twelve rounds per roll. Place on a baking sheet about 1/2 inches apart, and bake for 15 minutes.
6. Serve with mustards in various shape.

TEMPEH STUFFED CREMINI MUSHROOMS

Active Time: 15 minutes
Cook time: 20 minutes
Total Time: 35 minutes

Protein: 6 grams per serving (3 mushrooms)

Yield: 6 YIELD
A change on stuffed mushrooms here. In the filling, there is no bread or panko, but plenty of flavour together with rice and tempeh.

INGREDIENTS:

- 18 cremini mushrooms
- 2 table spoons of red onion, small dice
- 3 ounces tempeh, very thin diced or pulsed Pinch of onion powder Cayenne pepper 1/4 cup rice, fried
- 1 table spoon tamari

INSTRUCTIONS:

1. Cut from the mushrooms, and set aside the leaves. Chop the stems finely, then set aside.
2. In a small skillet melt 3 table spoons of water. Stir in the chopped stems of mushroom and onion. Stir in for 10 to 15 minutes or until transparent onion. Stir in the tempeh and simmer for another 5 minutes. Remove ground onion, cayenne pepper, corn, and tamari. Cook for 2 minutes, then stir occasionally.
3. Preheat to 350 ° F on burner.
4. Stuff the caps with mushroom and place them on the baking sheet. Bake for another 20 minutes.

ROASTED TACO-SEASONED EDAMAME AND CHICKPEAS

Active Time: 10 minutes
Cook time: 40 minutes
Total Time: 50 minutes

Protein: 7½ grams per serving (½ cup)

Yield: 7 YIELD

Get a little cup out and fill it with these spicy protein nibbles, which are easy to carry. They're baked to the perfect crispness and made to indulge on your day out.

INGREDIENTS:

- 12 ounces of frozen edamame
- 115-ounce can be used for chickpeas, drained (save the liquid to be used as aquafaba) and rinsed
- 4 teaspoons of taco seasoning
- 3 tablespoons of aquafaba.

INSTRUCTIONS

1. Preheat to 400 ° F on burner.
2. Cook the edamame on box according to instructions.
3. Place the chickpeas on a baking sheet, and prepare edamame. Bake for another 20 minutes.
4. Place the taco in a medium bowl to season.
5. Take the edamame from the oven and chickpeas, and mix with the aquafaba. Apply seasoning to taco bowl and paint well.
6. Go to the microwave, and bake 10 minutes more.
7. You can eat these as soon as they have cooled enough to handle, but before packing away, let them cool down in the oven for 2 hours to overnight. Keep in jar which is airtight. They are going to keep for 2 weeks.

SLOW COOKER SPICED PEANUTS

Active Time: 10 minutes
Cook time: 1 hour 15 minutes
Total Time: 1 hour 25 minutes
Yield: 6 YIELD

Protein: 19 grams per serving (½ cup)

Such peanuts are delicious and easy to make from slow cooker. People will think you've given them a lot of money, and they must have come in a lovely box.

INGREDIENTS:

- 3 cups peanuts
- 2 teaspoons extra virgin olive oil
- 1/2 teaspoon ground cumin
- 1/2 teaspoon garlic powder
- 1/2 teaspoon cayenne powder
- 1/2 teaspoon smoked paprika
- 1/2 teaspoon salt

INSTRUCTIONS:

1. Position the peanuts in a slow cooker. Add the oil and mix, so that all the peanuts have a little bit of oil. It'll suffice.

2. Pour in the seasoning and whisk. Cook for 1 hour at low. Uncover, and then cook for another 15 minutes.

MAPLE-GLAZED MIXED NUTS

Active Time: 5 minutes
Cook time: 15 minutes
Total Time: 20 minutes
Yield: 6 YIELD

Protein: 10 grams per serving (½ cup)

This protein snack is easy to make and only takes minutes. The outcome is maple-sweet candied nuts which would be a love present for anyone.

INGREDIENTS:

- 1 cup of walnuts
- 1 cup of pecans
- 1 cup of cashews
- 11/2 cups of maple syrup.

INSTRUCTIONS

Preheat to 325 ° F on oven.

2. In a medium bowl, mix the nuts and the maple syrup together. Make sure each nut is well coated. Spread out on a baking sheet, so that they are all connected to each other in one row. It's OK to contact. Bake for seven minutes.

3. Lift from the oven and turn a spatula open. Some at this stage, they will overlap. Put in the oven again and bake for another 6 minutes or so. Watch carefully. They start burning quickly if they are too long in.

4. Remove the baking sheet from the oven, open the nuts again and let it cool off completely. Eat or load straight away in an airtight container. These nuts will keep for quite a few weeks in your pantry, and will keep about 2 to 3 months in the fridge. These will be processed for 6 months by the fridge.

SPROUTED GRAIN TOAST WITH NUT BUTTER AND BANANA

Active Time: 10 minutes
Total Time: 10 minutes
Yield: 2 YIELD

Protein: 11 grams per serving

It's more of a how-to than a recipe, but if it's not published in a cookbook, you might forget it. And you wouldn't want to forget that. How can one taste so nice something so simple?

INGREDIENTS:

- 1/4 cup peanut butter
- 1/4 cup raw shelled hempseed
- 1 banana, cut

INSTRUCTIONS:

1. Toast bread. Split the angle in two. Layer the peanut butter with 2 teaspoons on each slice of toast.
2. Sprinkle the hempseed on top of each toast triangle and Banana sheet slices.

PEANUT BUTTER BANANA BREAKFAST COOKIES

Active Time: 10 minutes
Cook time: 25 minutes
Total Time: 35 minutes
Yield: 24 YIELD

Protein: 7¾ grams per serving (3 cookies)

The list of ingredients that make up these healthy protein cookies won't you believe. They are rustic in nature and pleasing in price.

INGREDIENTS:

- 2 bananas
- 1/3 cup of creamy peanut butter mashed
- 2/3 cup of unsweetened applesauce
- 1/4 cup almond flour
- 2 teaspoons of raw shelled hempseed
- 1 teaspoon vanilla extract
- 11/2 cups of fast-cooking oats
- 1/2 cup of pitted berries, sliced

INSTRUCTIONS:

1. Preheat to 350 ° F on burner.

2. Fill a parchment paper baking sheet, then set aside.
3. Stir in a large bowl with the mashed banana and peanut butter and blend well. Attach the applesauce, rice, cinnamon and hempseed. Blend well. Stir the dates and the oatmeal in.
4. Drop the cookie dough onto the prepared baking sheet, 1 heaping tablespoon at a time, about 2 inches apart. Flatten with fork back. 25 Minutes to bake cookies.
5. Remove from the oven and let the cookies cool for 5 minutes, then switch to a refrigerated rack.
Note: These cookies may also be freezed after baking. Pack in a freezer bag, and stack up to 6 months in the fridge. Add as many Breakfast Cookies as you like. At room temperature, they'll take around 30 minutes to defrost.

SEITAN LINKS TOFU SCRAMBLE

Active Time: 15 minutes
Cook time: 20 minutes
Total Time: 35 minutes
Yield: 6 YIELD

Protein: 29 grams per serving

One of the best ways to prepare tofu is through a scramble. Take it one step further and add some vegetables and seitan and you've got a big breakfast with food.

INGREDIENTS:

- 1 tablespoon of milk-free butter
- 1/2 cup of onion
- 8 ounces of mushrooms
- 16 ounces of extra firm tofu, peeled, pressed and crumbled
- 8 ounces Slow Cooker Maple Breakfast Links, cut thick
- 1 15 ounce of black beans, drained and rinsed

- 2 teaspoons of nutritional yeast
- 1/2 teaspoon of chili powder
- 1/2 teaspoon of paprika
- 1/2 teaspoon of black salt
- 1/2 teaspoon of turmeric
- 1/4 teaspoon In a broad skillet

INSTRUCTIONS

1. Heat up the butter over medium - high pressure. Add the connections between the onion, the mushrooms, tofu and seitan. Dredge 15 minutes.
2. Remove the black beans, nutritional yeast and all the seasonings and spices. Heat, and serve for 5 minutes.

BUCKWHEAT COCONUT PORRIDGE

Active Time: 15 minutes
Cook time: 10 minutes
Total Time: 25 minutes
Yield: 2 YIELD

Protein: 20 grams per serving

Here is your buckwheat using chance! In this compost Buckwheat is porridge. It's a great meal that will sustain you for a long time to come.

INGREDIENTS:

- 1 cup of smooth buckwheat cereal
- 1/2 tablespoon cinnamon
- 1/4 teaspoon salt
- 1/4 cup peanut butter
- 1/2 cup coconut cream
- 1/4 cup pecans
- 2 table spoons of fresh shelled hempseed

- 1/4 cup maple syrup

INSTRUCTIONS:

1. Put 3 tablespoons of water into a medium saucepan to simmer. Stir in the cereal, cinnamon, and salt. Reduce heat to low medium, then cover. Cook, stirring occasionally, for 8 minutes until all of the water is absorbed. Whisk in peanut butter and cream with coconut.
2. Serve with the cranberries, pecans, hempseed, and maple syrup in 2 containers and garnish.

SLOW COOKER APPLES AND OATS

Active Time: 15 minutes
Cook time: 3 hours
Total Time: 3 hours 15 minutes
Yield: 2 YIELD

Protein: 15 grams per serving

Here is a great meal that you will like again and again. This dish feeds two or three people but for a larger family it can be quickly doubled or tripled.

INGREDIENTS:

- 11/2 cups peeled and sliced apples
- 1 cup old-fashioned oats
  1/2 cup dairy-free butter, melted
- 1/2 cup coconut sugar
- 2 table lemon juice
- 2 table spoons hempseed, toasted in shell
- 1 tablespoon ground cinnamon
- 1 cup pecans, minced

INSTRUCTIONS:

1. Place all the ingredients in the slow cooker and mix. Turn up (it

has to cook on top). Cook for 2 to 3 hours, depending on the doneness you need. Serve dry, hot or cold.

OVERNIGHT MUESLI

Active Time: 15 minutes
Total Time: 15 minutes and then overnight
Yield: 6 YIELD

Protein: 15 grams per serving

Nighttime breakfasts aren't just for oats. Creating this recycle from homemade muesli is as simple as mixing ingredients in a bowl. It will keep for days as an extra bonus.

INGREDIENTS:

- 2 cups of old-fashioned oats
- 1 cup of raisins
- 1/2 cup of wheatgerm
- 1/2 cup of oat bran
- 1/2 cup of seeds
- 1/2 cup of pepitas
- 1/4 cup of wheat bran
- 1/4 cup of slivered almonds
- 1/4 cup of walnuts
- 1/4 cup of sunflower seed kernels
- 7 cups of almond milk or other egg free dairy

INSTRUCTIONS

1. Place all the dry substances in a large mixing bowl. Blend well. Pour in the milk again and stir well.
2. To stay overnight, cover and put in the refrigerator.
3. The muesli are ready to eat in the morning and will retain for 4 to 5 days.

ALL-IN-ONE SKILLET BREAKFAST HASH

Active Time: 15 minutes
Cook time: 25 minutes
Total Time: 40 minutes
Yield: 6 YIELD

Protein: 30 grams per serving

Here's a hardy breakfast that will feed a large group with satisfaction guaranteed. This will stick to your ribs, just as any good protein meal should.

INGREDIENTS

- 2 tablespoons coconut oil
- 2 cups diced russet potatoes
- 2 cups diced sweet potatoes
- 1 cup diced white onion
- 8 ounces extra-firm tofu, drained and pressed
- 2 teaspoons black salt
- 1½ teaspoons onion powder
- 1½ teaspoons garlic powder
- ½ teaspoon turmeric
- ½ teaspoon thyme
- ¼ teaspoon ground black pepper
- 2 cups Slow Cooker Maple Breakfast Links, sliced
- 2 tablespoons nutritional yeast

INSTRUCTIONS

1. In a very large skillet, either 12 inches wide or very deep, heat the oil over medium-high heat. Add the russet potatoes and cook for 10 minutes, flipping once. Add the sweet potatoes and onion; stir and cook 5 more minutes.
2. Push the potatoes and onions to the side and crumble the tofu into the pan. Add all of the spices and mix with the tofu. Cook 2 to 3 minutes or until you see that the turmeric is dispersed well and the tofu has turned a golden color.
3. Add the links and nutritional yeast and mix the whole skillet of

ingredients together. Cook 2 to 3 minutes or until the links are heated through. Taste and season with more salt and pepper, if desired.

MIXED PROTEIN ENCHILADA BREAKFAST

Active Time: 40 minutes
Cook time: 40 minutes
Total Time: 1 hour 20 minutes
Yield: 6 YIELD
Protein: 28 grams per serving

These cheesy enchiladas fill up enough for a huge weekend day and are complex enough to have a very satisfying breakfast or dinner. Tofu and seitan are both protagonists

INGREDIENTS:

Filling

- 11/4 cups Steamed Seitan Chipotle Links
- 11/2 cups broccoli flowers
- 1 table spoon coconut oil
- 4 ounces extra firm tofu, drained and pressed
- 1 table spoon nutritional yeast
- 11/2 teaspoon black salt
- 3/4 teaspoon ground black pepper
- 1/4 teaspoon turmeric
- 1/4 teaspoon paprika
- 1 15-ounce can pinto beans, drained and rinsed
- 1 teaspoon salt White Sauce 2 table

INSTRUCTIONS

1. Place the seitan bits in a food processor and spin until they crumble gently.
2. Add water with a steamer insert to a medium saucepan, and bring to a boil. Add the broccoli to the insert, and steam 10

minutes over boiling water. Remove, and set aside from the steamer.

3. Steam up the oil over medium to high heat in a large skillet. Crumble the tofu into your skillet and use your hands. Remove and cook for 3 minutes, breaking up any remaining too large pieces. Add the seeds, black salt, 1/2 teaspoon pepper, turmeric, and paprika. Stir to merge. Add the seitan, broccoli, beans, salt and 1/4 teaspoon pepper. Stir to combine. Replace, and set aside from the sun.

White Sauce

4. Melt the butter over medium to high heat into a medium saucepan. Add the flour, then stir and cook for 1 minute. Stir in the milk and carry to a low boil. Occasionally, whisk to avoid the lumps out of the sauce. Turn the heat to medium, and add salt and nutritional yeast. Stir and keep cooking to let it thicken a little bit. Replace, and set aside from the sun.

5. Preheat to 350 ° F on oven.

6. Add 3 tablespoons of enchilada sauce in a9-inch square, or 8-by-10-inch casserole dish. Constructed over the surface.

7. In the skillet split the filling into six parts. This can be eyeball or you can make creases in a pie shape when filling.

8. Lay a tortilla out and spread it lightly with enchilada sauce. Fill a sixth of the container with tofu. Roll up and put in a casserole platter. Continue to fill and rolle all six tortillas. Pour over the baked tortillas all of the leftover enchilada sauce.

9. When thickened, heat up the white sauce again, so you can spoon it over the top of the enchilada sauce. Cover for 30 minutes, then roast.

10. Uncover, garnish with olives, cilantro and green onions, and serve.

SEITAN BALLS WITH SLOW COOKER SPAGHETTI SAUCE
Active Time: 15 minutes
Cook time: 8 hours
Total Time: 8 hours 15 minutes
Yield: 6 YIELD

Protein: 27 grams per serving

This is one of those recettes made for by the slow cooker. The sauce is perfect on low and slow heating.

INGREDIENTS:

- 2 table spoons extra virgin olive oil
- 2 cups finely diced yellow onion
- 4 cloves garlic, finely diced
- 2 28-ounce cans diced tomatoes
- 46-ounce cans tomato paste
- 1 teaspoon crumbled bay leaf
- 2 table spoon coconut sugar
- 1 teaspoon oregano
- 1 teaspoon basil
- 1 teaspoon salt
- 1/2 teaspoon ground black pepper
- 11/2 cups Slow Cooker Versatile Seitan Balls
- 12 ounces spaghetti

INSTRUCTIONS:

1. Add the oil to a large skillet and heat up to reasonably high. Add the onion and sauté, for about 10 to 15 minutes, until translucent. Turn the heat down to medium and add the garlic and cook for another 2 minutes. Add all the ingredients to the slow cooker (except the seitan and pasta), plus 11/2 cups water. Cook at low for 6 to 8 hours, in the last hour adding the seitan. If you want to cook on fast, add the seitan for the last half hour, then cook 3 to 4

hours.
2. Cook the spaghetti according to the instructions of the box and eat with pasta sauce in seitan.

BAKED TOFU WITH SPICY TAHINI SAUCE

Active Time: 15 minutes
Cook time: 25 minutes
Total Time: 40 minutes
Yield: 4 YIELD

Protein: 20 grams per serving

When you're armed with this recipe there's no need for takeout. Baked tofu is dredged in a spicy sauce which can be whipped up instantly. You could be tempted to double that topping.

INGREDIENTS:

- 11/2 cups of jasmine rice
- 14 ounces of extra-firm tofu, soaked, pressed and sliced into 1/2-inch cubes
- 11/4 cup tahini
- 1/4 cup tamari
- 1/4 cup rice vinegar
- 1/4 cup maple syrup
- 1/2 teaspoon ground ginger
- 1 clove garlic, slimming
- 1/2 teaspoon sriracha Fresh thyme, for garnish (optional)

INSTRUCTIONS

1. Preheat to 400 ° F on burner. Fill a parchment-papered baking sheet.
2. In a saucepan add the rice and cover with 3 cups of water. Cover, bring boil and turn heat down. Cook covered for about 15 minutes

or until it consumes water.
3. Place the tofu cubes on the baking sheet packed, and bake for 15 minutes. Flip with a spatula, and cook 10 minutes longer. Deposit back.
4. Make the sauce whilst the tofu is baking: add tahini, tamari, 1/2 cup water, rice vinegar, maple syrup, ginger, garlic, and sriracha to a cup. Mix well, and heat until creamy and hot.
5. Stir in ready tofu and serve hot over rice. If needed, garnish with a thyme.

STUFFED SWEET POTATOES WITH TAHINI DRESSING
Active Time: 20 minutes
Cook time: 1 hour
Total Time: 1 hour 20 minutes
Yield: 2 YIELD

Protein: 34 grams per serving

This food in one pretty package makes a complete dinner. Sweet and savory aromas are served together, then slathered as a foil with the perfect dressing.

INGREDIENTS:
Sweet Potatoes and Stuffing

- 2 sweet potatoes
- 1 tablespoon of coconut oil
- 1/4 cup of white onion
- 4 ounces of white mushrooms, sliced
- 1 cup of Slow Cooker Versatile Seitan Balls, chopped
- 1/4 teaspoon of ground cumin
- 1/4 teaspoon of onion powder
- 1/4 teaspoon of salt Pinch of ground black pepper

Tahini

- 1/4 cup of tahini
- 1 tablespoon of maple syrup
- 1 tablespoon of lemon juice
- 1 clove of garlic
- 1/4 teaspoon of salt

INSTRUCTIONS

1.Preheat to 350 ° F on burner.

2. In the preheated oven put the sweet potatoes and bake for 40 to 45 minutes or until tender.

3. Meanwhile, heat over medium - high heat and add the oil to a large skillet. Attach the mushrooms and onion, and sauté for 10 minutes. Remove the seitan, cumin, onion powder, salt and pepper and continue cooking for another 5 minutes. Deposit back.

4. Cut the top off the sweet potatoes ' long side, and pick out the cores the best you can. Put the centers in a bowl to medium. Remove from skillet to bowl all but 1/3 cup of the seitan-mushroom mixture. Blend well. Stuff the combination of sweet potatoes back into the containers. Put back into the oven at 350 ° F for 15 minutes to heat up.

Sauce tahini

5. Mix all the ingredients of the tahini sauce together with 3 table spoons of water during this time. Deposit back.

6. Take the potatoes from the oven, and put them on a serving platter. Drizzle the tahini sauce over the stuffed sweet potatoes and scatter on top of the rest of the seitan-mushroom mixture.

VEGAN THREE-BEAN PASTA WITH CREAMY SPINACH SAUCE

Active Time: 10 minutes

Cook time: 40 minutes

Total Time: 50 minutes

Yield: 6 YIELD

Protein: 8 grams per serving

A healthy high-protein vegan pasta recipe, perfect for vegetarians, with 17 grams of protein per serving of all those beans, plus plenty of nutrients and fibre. This pasta recipe combines three types of beans with spinach in a healthy vegan white sauce.

INGREDIENTS

- 1 tablespoon of olive oil
- 1 large (sliced) onion
- 2 cloves of garlic (crushed)
- 1 red bell pepper (cut)
- 1 teaspoon of dried oregano
- 1 15-ounce can cut tomatoes, or 2 cups of fresh tomatoes
- 1/2 cup of cooked red kidney beans
- 1/2 cup of cooked navy beans
- 1/2 cup of cooked chickpeas
- 1 cup of cooked pasta tubes
- 2 tablespoons of margarine
- 4 tablespoons of fresh chickpeas

INSTRUCTIONS

1. Steam up the oil over medium heat in a large saucepan. Cook the onion, garlic, and pepper gently until the vegetables are tender, about 8 minutes.
2. Add the chickpeas, onions, beans, and oregano. Season with salt and pepper, to taste. Cover and boil the saucepan for 20 minutes.
3. Prepare the pasta as indicated by box. Drain and add to the mixture of cooked beans and place this mixture in a shallow serving dish.
4. Heat the margarine over medium heat in a medium saucepan to form the sauce. Stir in the rice, and add the soy milk slowly. Stir constantly to a simmer and cook for 2 to 3 minutes, then season

with the nutmeg and salt and pepper.
5. Heat the spinach for 5 minutes in 2 table spoons of water. Thoroughly drain, and add to the sauce. Remove to well blended.
6. Pour the bean mixture over sauce and serve immediately.

CHICKPEA SEITAN FRIED RICE

Active Time: 15 minutes
Cook time: 15 minutes
Total Time: 30 minutes
Yield: 2 YIELD

Protein: 40 grams per serving

You're not going to break a sweat over this recipe. A little cooking and boiling in a pan unites all the flavors in no time.

INGREDIENTS:

- 1 cup jasmine rice
- 1 cup Pressure Cooker Tender Patties
- 115-ounce can chickpeas, drained and rinsed
- 3 table spoons tamari
- 3 table spoons maple syrup
- 1/4 teaspoon ground ginger
- 2 table spoon coconut oil
- 2 carrots, peeled and diced small
- 1 clove garlic, minced green onions, trimmed, for garnish

INSTRUCTIONS:

1. Add the rice and remove 2 cups of water to a medium saucepan. Bring to a boil, cover, turn heat down to low, and simmer for 20 minutes or until the water is consumed and the rice is tender. Deposit back.
2. Place the seitan in a food processor, and spin to make small bits a few times. Turn into a tub.
3. Add the chickpeas to the food processor and pulse them, about three or four pulses, to make small pieces.

4. In a small bowl, add the tamari, maple syrup, and ginger and set aside.
5. Add the oil and heat to a large skillet over medium - high heat. Attach the carrots and fry with a spatula, tossing for about 5 to 10 minutes. Turn the heat down to prevent the carrots from frying, if necessary. Cook for 1 minute, add the garlic and stir; Add the rice, chickpeas prepared and seitan and start to sauté until the seitan has some browning. Add the sauce mixture and continue to stir and flip with a spatula to incorporate all the sauce and to cook it slightly.
6. Garnished serving with sliced green onions.

YOGHURT WITH APPLES, ALMONDS AND CHIA SEEDS

Active Time: 5 minutes
Cook Time: 5 minutes
Total Time: 10 minutes
YIELD: 1

Protein: 6 grams per serving

INGREDIENTS

- 150 g of natural yogurt
- 1 apple
- 1 - 2 tablespoons chopped almonds
- 1 teaspoon honey (at will)
- 1 teaspoon chia seeds (alternatively flax seeds)

INSTRUCTIONS

1. The almonds are roasted in a pan and then set aside to cool. Quarter the apple, free from the core and cut into small cubes. The shell can stay calm.
2. The yoghurt is then mixed with the apples, almonds, and honey and chia seeds.

CHIA BERRY GREEN SMOOTHIE

Active Time: 5 minutes
Cook Time: 5 minutes
Total Time: 10 minutes
YIELD: 2

Protein: 16 grams per serving

INGREDIENTS

- 2 cups of spinach
- 1 1/2 cup of water
- 1 orange (peeled)
- 1 cup of strawberry
- 1 cup blueberry (frozen)
- 2 tablespoons chia seed

INSTRUCTIONS

1 . Add spinach, water and chia seeds to the mixer. Mix until smooth.

3. Add the remaining ingredients and blend again. pleasant!

CHIA SEED WITH FRESH VEGETABLE JUICE

Active Time: 5 minutes
Cook Time: 10 minutes
Total Time: 15 minutes
YIELD: 5

Protein: 14 grams per serving

INGREDIENTS

- 1 pineapple unit
- 5 tablespoons Chia Seed dessert
- 3 units of green apple
- 300 milliliters of orange juice
- 1 pinch of Stevia or sweetener

INSTRUCTIONS

1 .Take the orange and pineapple juice without a heart in a bowl in a bowl and blend very well until the ingredients are integrated.

2. Wash the apples and add them in medium squares where we have the preparation of the previous step to continue making our pineapple and chia smoothie. Blend or process until all ingredients are integrated.

3. Finally, add stevia powder (a pinch) to give a sweet touch to our shake to lose weight. This step is not mandatory, the fruit already has natural sugars and there is no need to add extra, but if you think the flavor is very strong we recommend using sweeteners or honey.

4. Once all the ingredients have been liquefied, add the chia seeds to each of the glasses where we will serve the smoothies.

Serve pineapple and chia juice to lose weight decorating with seeds. It is ideal that this juice is taken in the morning, taking into account the fruits it contains, it serves as a diuretic and for people who have problems with their digestive system.

VEGETARIAN GOULASH

Active Time: 20 minutes
Cook Time: 50 minutes
Total Time: 1 hour 10 minutes
YIELD: 4

Protein: 8 grams per serving

INGREDIENTS

- 1Pk Tofu (smoked)
- 500g sauerkraut
- 2 Cup Soup
- 1 onion
- 3 Garlic cloves
- 3 olive oil
- 3 tomato paste
- 3 Caraway seed
- 2 paprika
- salt and pepper
- 1 shot vinegar
- 1 cup creme fraiche

INSTRUCTIONS

1. For the vegetarian goulash, first peel the onion and garlic and chop. Dice tofu into bite-size pieces.
2. Sauté the onion, garlic and tofu in a saucepan with a little oil, Stir in the tomato paste and steam briefly. Now add the sauerkraut and pour in the soup.
3. The goulash is seasoned with paprika powder and caraway and should now simmer for 50 minutes.
4. Finally stir in creme fraiche and season with salt, pepper and vinegar. Let it sit briefly and serve.

FRIED RICE RECIPE

Active Time: 30 minutes
Cook Time: 45 minutes
Total Time: 1 hour15 minutes
YIELD: 4

Protein: 10 grams per serving

INGREDIENTS

- 1 cup basmati or other rice
- 2 carrots
- piece of Italian cabbage
- 3 stalks of celery
- 2 spring onions
- 4 garlic cloves
- 2 tablespoons soy sauce or tamari
- 2 tbsp sesame
- 2 tbsp oil
- 2 eggs (optional) or ½ tofu cubes
- salt and spices to taste

INSTRUCTIONS

1. Break eggs, salt and beat them. Mix with soy sauce. If you don't use eggs, mash the tofu with a fork and mix with soy sauce.
2. Heat oil, put carrots in a frying pan for 1 minute, add celery, chopped cabbage and spring onion after a while.
3. After 3 minutes, put in the rice and fry until it is hot. Pour the eggs and stir them vigorously to make them stick to the rice. Sprinkle with sesame seeds and serve warm.

BUTTERNUT PUMPKIN VEGAN TOFU LASAGNA

Active Time: 25 minutes
Cook Time: 1 hour
Total Time: 1 hour 25 minutes
YIELD: **4**

Protein: 18 grams per serving

INGREDIENTS

- 2 pack (14 ounces) extra farm tofu, drained
- 4 tablespoons of nutrient yeast
- 1.5 tablespoons of Italian seasoning (or 1 teaspoon of oregano, basil, parsley)
- 2 tsp garlic powder
- Salt and pepper
- 1 tablespoon extra virgin olive oil
- Chopped onion
- 1 chopped garlic
- 1 medium-sized pumpkin
- 3 bell peppers diced
- one bottle (40 oz) marinara sauce

INSTRUCTIONS

1. Grease the oven and heat the firstly to 400 degrees. Wrap the tofu with a thin kitchen towel (or paper towel) and press firmly to drain the tofu. Repeat until you have as much tofu as much as needed.
2. With a big bowl in view, mix the tofu while you crush it with a fork until it breaks. Add nutritive yeast, Italian seasoning, garlic and season with salt and pepper. I'll save it.
3. Cut out the bulbous end of the pumpkin and reserve it for future use. Take the neck and first cut the top and peel it off.
4. Cut the pumpkin in half vertically, taking care not to penetrate the center. Swirl the pumpkin around blade A. Set the pumpkin slice aside.
5. Heat the oil with medium high heat in a medium pan. When the oil shines, add onions, garlic and chili and cook for about 5 minutes until soft and crisp.

6. Add marinara sauce and cook for another 5 minutes to heat the sauce.

GOURMET VEGETARIAN TABBOULEH SALAD WITH EDAMAME AND FETA

Active time: 35 minutes
Cook time: 0 minutes
Total time: 35 minutes
Protein: 10 grams per serving

Yield: 4

If you like conventional vegetarian tobbouleh salad, try this gourmet tobbouleh made with feta and edamame soya. This is an unusual and delicious vegetarian tabbouleh dish, filled with pesto and fresh herbs for plenty of flavour. Delish: Delish!

INGREDIENTS

- 1 1/4 cups of uncooked bulgur wheat
- 2 cups of water, boil
- 1/4 cup of pesto prepared
- 3 tbsp. Fresh lemon juice
- 2 cups of cherry tomatoes, diced
- 3/4 cup (3 ounces) of feta , crumbled
- 1 15-ounce can of chickpeas, drained
- 1/3 cup of green onions (scallions), cut know
- 2 tbsp. New, minced parsley,
- 1/4 tsp. Freshly ground black pepper

INSTRUCTIONS

Guidelines for 2 cups shelled edamame

1. Combine the bulgur wheat and a large bowl of boiling water. Cover 30 minutes and let stand. Dump and dump.
2. Combine lemon juice and pesto; stir with whisk. In a large bowl, combine bulgur, pesto mixture, tomatoes, feta, chickpea, green onions, parsley, pepper, and edamame; and gently toss to combine.

Serve with half pita.

KALE AND FRISEE SALAD WITH SHERRY VINAIGRETTE

Active Time: 20 minutes
Cook Time: 60 minutes
Total Time: 1 hour 20 minutes
YIELD: **8**

Protein: 6 grams per serving

INGREDIENTS

- 1/4 cup extra virgin olive oil
- 3 tablespoons, drain and dab to dry
- 1/2 cup chopped roasted hazelnut
- 1 celery heart (pale center stem and leaves), chopped (about 1 cup)
- 1 1/2 teaspoon whole grain or stone powder mustard
- 2 tablespoons Sherry vinegar
- Kosher salt and freshly ground pepper
- Roughly chopped one head freeze (about 4 cups)
- Remove a small bunch of latinate kale, stalks and central rib bones and make them fine (about 4 cups)

INSTRUCTIONS

1. Heat two tablespoons of oil through an average heat in a small skillet. Add capers when oil shimmers. Cook until they swell and darken slightly, 1 1/2 to 2 minutes, stirring a few times. Attach the hazelnuts and cook for another 1 minute. Move the mixture to a small bowl (with oil). Let it cool, then whisk in the celery.
2. Alternatively, whisk together the mustard and vinegar in a large bowl. In the remaining 2 tablespoons of oil, slowly whisk to make

the dressing; sprinkle with salt. Remove frisée and kale, tossing to cover evenly; let stand for a total of 20 minutes and 1 hour. When served, finish with caper mixture.

HEARTY COTTAGE SPREAD ON WHOLEMEAL BREAD

Active Time: 10 minutes
Cook time: 10 minutes
Total time: 20 minutes
Serving: 2

Protein: 6 grams per serving

INGREDIENTS

- ¼ bar leek
- 1 carrot
- ½ tl mustard seeds
- 1 handful parsley
- 200 g cottage spread (10% fat in dry matter)
- salt
- 4 slices whole grain bread

INSTRUCTIONS

1. Clean leek, wash and cut into fine rings. Clean carrot, wash and finely grate. Mustard seed pounded with a mortar. Wash parsley, shake dry and chop.

2. Mix cottage spread, leek, carrot and mustard together and season with salt. Spread the bread with the spread and sprinkle with the parsley.

FRIED QUINOA
Active Time: 10 minutes
Cook Time: 20 minutes
Total Time: 30 minutes
YIELD: **5**

Protein: 10 grams per serving

INGREDIENTS

- 1 cup of quinoa
- 1 cup and a half water chicken soup or vegetable better and flavor
- ¼ minced onion
- 2 carrots peeled and chopped
- 3 chopped green onions
- 3 garlic cloves
- Chopped fresh raw ginger 1/2 teaspoon
- 1 tablespoon olive oil
- 2 beaten eggs
- ½ cup thawed beans
- For source:
- 1 tablespoon and half of teriyaki sauce
- 2 tablespoons soy sauce
- ¾ teaspoon sesame oil

INSTRUCTIONS

1. Clean the quinoa in cold water several times to absorb the saponin.
2. Take the quinoa and the water to a boil in a small saucepan, then reduce to a cooler. Season to taste with salt.
3. Simmer until the quinoa is ready for 15-20 minutes, doubling in volume and releasing the white germ.
4. Remove from heat and let stand for approximately five minutes. Let it cool down.
5. In a small bowl, combine the teriyaki sauce with soy sauce and sesame oil. Please book later.
6. Put half a spoonful of olive oil over high temperature in a large skillet. Add the onion and carrot and cook for about two minutes. Add to the pan the chopped scallions, garlic and ginger. Cook two more minutes.
7. Add the remaining olive oil and quinoa. Sauté about two minutes. Add the sauce and saute another two minutes.
8. Make a hole in the centre of the quinoa to pour the eggs and peas and stir until the desired presentation.

WHOLEGRAIN BASMATI RICE WITH CRUNCHY VEGETABLES AND ALMONDS

Active Time: 10 minutes
Cook Time: 35 minutes
Total Time: 45 minutes
YIELD: 2

Protein: 12 grams per serving

INGREDIENTS

- 200 grams whole grain basmati rice
- 400ml water

- 1 pinch salt
- 1 broccoli
- 8th mini tomato
- 0.5 red pepper
- 6 brown mushrooms
- 2 tablespoons
- Almond (organic)
- Almond leaves
- 3 tablespoons
- Extra virgin olive oil
- Black pepper
- salt

INSTRUCTIONS

1. Wash the rice thoroughly with colander.
2. Put twice the amount of water and a pinch of salt in the pan and soak for about 10 minutes. Boil at the highest heat setting, then boil at the lowest heat until the water has evaporated (about 30 minutes). Inflate with the lid closed.
3. Wash broccoli and divide into small florets. Boil for a few minutes in a hot pot and then cool. Meanwhile, wash the tomato and pepper, cut the pepper into small pieces and cut the tomato in half. Clean the mushrooms and slice them as well. Rinse the herbs and shake to dry.
4. Heat the oil in a large pan, fry almonds and vegetables, add broccoli and cook well. Season with pepper, salt and basil
5. Serve

BROCCOLI POTATO CASSEROLE

Active Time: 45 minutes
Cook Time: 45 minutes
Total Time: 1 hour 30 minutes

YIELD: 4

Protein: 16 grams per serving

INGREDIENTS

- 750 g Potato
- 150 g Peas, frozen
- 300 g broccoli
- 2 garlic
- 30 g butter
- 30 g Flour
- 600 mlmilk
- 2 bay leaves
- salt and pepper
- 100 g cooked ham

INSTRUCTIONS

1. Wash the potatoes and cook them as boiled potatoes in salt water. Thawed peas. Clean the broccoli, divide it into small flowers, peel the stems and slice them. Drain the potatoes, stir-fry, peel and cut into slices about 1/2 cm thick. Peel garlic and cut into thin slices.
2. Melt butter in a pan and fry garlic. Add flour and stir while stirring. Deglaze with milk Bring to a boil, add bay leaf, season with salt and pepper, simmer for 10 minutes on low heat and stir several times. Remove bay leaf and season with salt, pepper.
3. Finely grind Italian hard potatoes. Cut the ham into strips. Mix potatoes, broccoli, peas, ham, 100 g gouda and gravy. Put in a casserole dish and sprinkle with the rest of Gouda. Bake in a 200 ° (convection 180 °) hot oven in the center rack for 40-45 minutes.

ALMONDS AND BARLEY PILAF

Active Time: 20 minutes
Cook Time: 60 minutes
Total Time: 1 hour 20 minutes
YIELD: 8

Protein: 20 grams per serving

INGREDIENTS

- 1 C. (300 g) uncooked barley, brown rice, Faro, or burger
- 2 1/2 C. (625 ml) water or broth
- 2-4 T. Olive oil (split)
- 1 C. (100-150 g) coarsely chopped almonds, walnuts, or pecans
- 1 finely chopped onion
- 8-10 C of raw vegetables such as celery, carrot, zucchini, summer pumpkin, broccoli, peppers, cauliflower, fennel, mushrooms

INSTRUCTIONS

1. In a container filled with salty water cook barley for 45 minutes or thereabout. you may cook the Barley the previous day before making pilaf.
2. Heat 1T.using the frying pan, add and fry the nuts until color becomes light brown.
3. Using a frying pan, use 3T. olive oil to fry preferred vegetable until its tender. it does not matter if you have different type of vegetable added together
4. Stir cooked barley and nuts in a vegetable mixture and heat before serving.

RED LENTIL AND VEGETABLE STEW

Active Time: 25 minutes
Cook Time: 20 minutes
Total Time: 45 minutes
YIELD: **4**

Protein: 10 grams per serving

INGREDIENTS

- 1 Onion
- 2 Carrot
- 2 Potato
- 3 pole/s celery
- 2 tbsp oil
- 1 liter vegetable stock
- 2 tbsp tomato paste
- 250 g Lentils, red
- 1 teaspoon curry powder
- 1 Bay leaf
- 1 tbsp Aceto balsamico
- 1 tbsp Ketchup
- salt and pepper
- sour cream
- Parsley, chopped

INSTRUCTIONS

1. Dice the onion and vegetables, wash the lentils. Brown the onions in a large saucepan in oil, add the vegetables and the curry powder and briefly fry the tomato paste.
2. Then deglaze with the vegetable broth, add the bay leaf and bring the broth to a boil. After about 5 minutes of cooking, add the

lentils and cook for another 10 minutes. Should the stew become too firm, add some vegetable stock.
3. Finally, with aceto balsamic vinegar, ketchup and maybe some pepper, salt and curry to taste. Bring out the bay leaf.
4. Serve the stew in plates, eg with a dollop of sour cream and fresh parsley. Serve with bread.

SAVOY CABBAGE AND APPLE VEGETABLES WITH RED LENTILS AND DATES

Active Time: 30 minutes
Cook Time: 10 minutes
Total Time: 40 minutes
YIELD: 2

Protein: 20 grams per serving

INGREDIENTS

- 1 shallot
- 400 g savoy
- 200 g sour apples (1 sour apple)
- 50 g dried date (without stone)
- 2 tbsp olive oil
- 100 g red lenses
- 150 ml classic vegetable broth
- salt
- pepper
- 50 g hazelnuts
- 50 g rocket (0.5 bunch)

INSTRUCTIONS

1. Peel the shallot and finely chop.

2. Clean the savoy cabbage, remove the hard stalk, wash, drain and cut into thin strips.
3. Wash apple, rub dry, quarter, core and dice. Halve dates, stone and cut into strips.
4. Heat oil in a large non-stick pan, Sauté the shallot briefly in a glass, add savoy cabbage and steam for about 5 minutes. Stir in apple, lentils and dates and cook over medium heat for another 2 minutes.
5. Add broth and simmer for another 10 minutes. Season with salt and pepper.
6. While cooking the savoy cabbage, roughly chop the hazelnuts and fry in a small frying pan until they start to smell fragrant. Remove from heat.
7. Clean the rocket, wash, shake dry and chop. Sprinkle with the hazelnuts over the vegetables and serve.

LENTIL AND VEGETABLE STEW

Active Time: 15 minutes
Cook Time: 60 minutes
Total Time: 1 hour 15 minutes
YIELD: 6

Protein: 12 grams per serving

INGREDIENTS

- 2 tablespoons olive oil
- 1 large onion, finely diced
- 2 tablespoons tomato paste
- 1 teaspoon dry time

- 1 piece of finely chopped garlic
- 3 celery stems, finely diced
- 3 carrots, peeled and finely diced
- 2 cups (12 ounces) of small green French lentils
- 8 cups of water or vegetable stock
- 1 tablespoon low sodium soy sauce
- 1 1/2 teaspoon salt
- 1/8 teaspoon pepper
- 3 tablespoons of lemon juice
- 1/2 bundle kale, with stem, sliced thinly, sideways

INSTRUCTIONS

1. Through the medium of heat add oil. Once the oil has sparkled, cook with onion and stir occasionally for 10 minutes or until deep golden.
2. Onions at the bottom of the lentil soup pot. Caramelized onion and tomato paste at the bottom of the soup pot.
3. Cook the tomato paste and vegetables: push the onion into the side of the pan and add tomato paste to the created space. Stir for 2-3 minutes or until the tomato paste is dark brown. Add thyme, garlic, celery, carrots. Cook and stir for 2 minutes.
4. Caramelized onion and tomato paste at the bottom of the soup pot. Caramelized onion and tomato paste at the bottom of the soup pot.
5. Boil the soup: add lentils, 8 cups of water, soy sauce, salt and pepper to the pan. Adjust to medium heat so that the soup can be boiled gently. Cook for 55-60 minutes
6. Finish the soup: Scoop out 2 cups of soup and puree with a blender until smooth, or use a soaking blender and puree to get the soup a little thicker on the body, but puree until the texture remains soft. Return the mixed soup to the pan and add lemon juice. Add the sliced kale and simmer for 1-2 minutes or until the kale is soft.
7. Add salt, pepper and lemon juice as you like. Serve with a nice

slice of crusty bread or side salad.

TEMPEH CHILI

Active Time: 10 minutes
Cook Time: 40 minutes
Total Time: 50 minutes
YIELD: **6**

Protein: 6 grams per serving

INGREDIENTS

- 2 tablespoons olive oil
- 8 ounce tempeh, diced
- 2 teaspoons soy sauce
- 1 red bell pepper, chopped
- 1 bell pepper, chopped
- 2 pieces of garlic, chopped
- 1 diced onion
- Canned 4 ounce sliced green chili
- 15 ounces of kidney beans or chili
- 8 ounce canned diced tomatoes
- 1 tablespoon chili powder
- 1/2 teaspoon cumin powder
- 1/4 teaspoon cayenne pepper, or taste

INSTRUCTIONS

1. Using a tablespoon of olive oil, fry the tempeh until it is golden (about 3-5 minutes). Then add the soy sauce and stir for 1-2 minutes until the soy sauce is sticky and melts. I'll save it.
2. In a large soup or stock pot, fry the onion, garlic, and bell pepper with the remaining olive oil until soft.
3. Add the rest of the **INGREDIENTS** except the coriander and

tempe with reduced heat
4. Simmer for at least 20 minutes up to 40 minutes, stir occasionally and add a little more liquid as needed.
5. Sprinkle with freshly chopped coriander.

PEANUT-BUTTER CINNAMON TOAST

Active Time: 10 minutes
Cook Time: 10 minutes
Total Time: 20 minutes
YIELD: **2**

Protein: 15 grams per serving

INGREDIENTS

- 90 g of butter at room temperature
- 2.5 tablespoons cinnamon powder
- 2 tablespoons brown sugar
- 2 slices of bread
- A pinch of salt

INSTRUCTIONS

1. Although it is as easy to prepare as any other, cinnamon toast requires a little preparation. In addition, we will dispense with the toaster to cook them directly on a nonstick skillet.
2. First of all, mix the 90 g of butter with the two and a half tablespoons of cinnamon and the two tablespoons of brown sugar.
3. Although the latter can be reduced if you are not very sweet tooth, It has to be homogeneous in both color and texture.
4. The best way to do this is to have the butter at room temperature , since if it is cold it will be almost impossible. I do not recommend that you microwave it, since if it melts it will not work for the recipe.

5. Once we have the cinnamon butter ready, it is time to spread it generously on both sides of the bread. Although anyone is worth it, my recommendation is to use a thick bread . If you prefer you can also use a loaf of bread
6. Finally, we put the nonstick skillet on the fire and toast the slices on both sides. It is not necessary to add oil, since the butter will ensure that it does not stick.
7. As for the temperature, it is best to start over high heat and then lower it a bit to prevent burning.
8. Once the cinnamon toast is browned they are ready to eat, although before spreading it in the coffee I recommend you to add a pinch of salt.

RAW PAPAYA AND CARROT SALAD

Active Time: 5 minutes
Cook Time: 10 minutes
Total Time: 15 minutes
YIELD: 4

Protein: 6 grams per serving

INGREDIENTS

- 200 g of green papaya
- Carrot 120 g
- Raw green beans 120 g
- Dried shrimp 120 g.
- Tomato 80 g
- 4 garlic cloves
- 40 g bird pepper (or not)
- Lemon juice 120g

- 60 g palm sugar (or brown sugar)
- 80 g tamarind paste (optional)
- 2 tablespoons peanuts to decorate

INSTRUCTIONS

1. Crush pepper and garlic. Cut green beans into 2 cm and cut tomatoes into quarters. Add lemon juice and coconut sugar and tamarind paste to this seasoning.
2. Peel and carrot carrots and papaya, add to previous INSTRUCTIONS. Finish by adding crushed or whole peanuts and dried shrimp.
3. Add carrot sticks and cucumber slices, carrot sticks and beans as needed.
4. Mix and serve ready

MAPLE CINNAMON BREAKFAST QUINOA

Active Time: 25 minutes
Cook Time: 20 minutes
Total Time: 45 minutes
YIELD: 2

Protein: 11 grams per serving

1. In this basic quinoa breakfast dish, the syrup, cinnamon and raisin flavors are common enough for children to eat it right up. Add whatever fruit you have on hand-bananas, strawberries, or berries are perfect. If you don't have time in the morning to cook quinoa, cook it the night before, or try using quinoa flakes that are easy to prepare.

This quinoa porridge breakfast meal is vegetarian, dairy, high protein and gluten-free.

INGREDIENTS:

- 1 cup quinoa
- 2 to 2 1/2 cups
- 2/3 cup soy milk
- 1 tsp water.
- 1/2 tsp vegan margarine.
- 2 Tbsp cinnamon.
- Additional maple syrup: 2 tbsp. Raisins Optional:
- 2 (sliced) bananas instructions

INSTRUCTIONS

1. Heat up the quinoa and bring the water to a boil in a small saucepan. Reduce to a simmer until the liquid is absorbed and allow to cook, covered, for 15 minutes.
2. Cook quinoa Take the quinoa off heat and fluff it with a fork. Cover, and give five minutes to settle in.
3. Fluff quinoa with a fork Stir in the margarine and soy milk, then the ingredients remaining.
4. Stir in the remaining ingredients and drink!

VEGAN TOFU SCRAMBLE WITH SPINACH

Active Time: 5 minutes
Cook Time: 10 minutes
Total Time: 15 minutes
YIELD: 2

Protein: 12 grams per serving

A spinach tofu scramble is very tasty and is the perfect breakfast protein boost for veggans wanting to start their day with an egg-like dish. The tofu is crumbled and then saute to resemble scrambled eggs— when combined with tomatoes, onions, mushrooms and spinach, you may not even know that you're not consuming chickens.

INGREDIENTS

- 2 teaspoons of olive oil
- 2 tomatoes (cut)
- 2 cloves of garlic (minced)
- 3/4 cup of sliced fresh mushrooms
- 1 bunch (10 ounces) of spinach (rinsed)
- 1 pound of firm or extra-firm tofu (well pressed and crumbled)
- 1/2 teaspoon of soy sauce
- 1 teaspoon of freshly squeezed lemon juice
- salt and pepper.

INSTRUCTIONS

1. Collect ingredients.
2. Heat the olive oil in a skillet and saute the tomatoes, garlic, and mushrooms for 2 to 3 minutes over medium heat.
3. Reduce heat to medium-low and add spinach, tofu crumbled, soy sauce, and juice lemon. Cover, stirring occasionally, and cook for 5 to 7 minutes.
4. Sprinkle, before eating, with salt and pepper.
5. Serve, and have fun!

FULL VEGAN APPLE PANCAKES

Active Time: 10 minutes
Cook Time: 10 minutes
Total Time: 20 minutes
YIELD: 4

Protein: 8 grams per serving

Apple pancakes in Vegan? Even better still! There's no need to skimp when it comes to food, just because you are vegetarian or vegan! Apple pecan pancakes are good, high in protein and sugar, made with soy milk and a bit of tofu, and taste positively scrumptious. This apple pecan pancakes recipe is vegetarian as well as vegan, making it egg-free and dairy-free too.

INGREDIENTS

- 1 1/2 cups of soy milk (or another vegan milk alternative
- 1/2 cup tofu (soft / silk)
- 1/3 cup shortening of vegetables
- 1 1/2 cups of flour
- 2 1/2 teaspoons of baking powder
- 1/2 teaspoon of salt
- 1/2 teaspoon of cinnamon
- 1/2 teaspoon of nutmeg
- 2 apples (cut)
- 1/3 cup of pecans (cut)
- 2 table spoons of oil (more or less as required for frying)

INSTRUCTIONS

1. Pulse all ingredients together in a blender or food processor except pecans until the apples are minced and the ingredients are mixed. You can also finely chop the apples by hand, and combine the ingredients together.
2. Fold in the pecans, gently.
3. Drop on a slightly oiled skillet or griddle with large spoonfuls and cook for a couple of minutes until bubbles appear. Flip and cook until golden brown is light on both sides.
4. Serve, and have fun!

VEGETARIAN LASAGNA

Active Time: 5 minutes
Cook Time: 10 minutes
Total Time: 15 minutes
YIELD: 2

Protein: 10 grams per serving

INGREDIENTS

- An eggplant
- A small zucchini.
- A carrot.
- 1/2 onion
- Half red pepper

Fried tomato, I personally like to buy it crushed and fry it myself by adding onion, basil, oregano, etc.

INSTRUCTIONS

1.Cut the eggplant into slices of about 3-4 millimeters. We put them in the microwave for 1 minute so they are cooked.
2. Chop the onion, zucchini, and red pepper and grate the carrot (I prefer to grate it to take less time to make it) and sauté everything well with a drizzle of olive oil.
3. When we have the sofrito ready we add a few tablespoons of tomato.
4. We assemble the lasagna: first we put a slice of eggplant, a spoonful or two of vegetables, another layer of eggplant, more vegetables and topping

When the lasagna is mounted, we put it in the microwave for 30 seconds to melt.

QUINOA SALAD WITH FRESH MINT AND PARSLEY RECIPE

Active Time: 15 minutes
Cook Time: 0 minutes
Total Time: 15 minutes
YIELD: 4

Protein: 10 grams per serving

Whole grain quinoa seasoned with fresh herbs, including fresh mint, parsley, lemon juice, and green onions, makes this salad recipe healthy and low fat, as well as vegetarian and vegan. Don't let that scare you – it also tastes good and just bursts with a lot of fresh flavour!

INGREDIENTS

- 2 cups quinoa (precooked)
- 1/2 cup pecans (can be substituted for pine nuts or almonds)
- 3 tbsp. Clean (cut) spinach
- 1/2 cup (cut) fresh parsley
- 3 scallions / green onions, (cut)
- 3 tbsp. Olive oil
- 2 centimetres. 1 tsp lemon juice.
- Garlic salt
- salt and pepper (to taste)

INSTRUCTIONS

1. Combine the quinoa, almonds, parsley, and mint in one large bowl.
2. Whisk the olive oil, lemon juice, and garlic salt together in a separate bowl, then spill over the precooked quinoa. Gently toss this dressing and the quinoa together to disperse evenly and combine well.
3. Season with ample salt and pepper
4. Place your quinoa salad in the fridge and allow to cool down for at least 15 minutes before serving to allow the flavors to blend.
5. Throw again gently before eating, and sample to see if more salt and pepper are needed; adjust seasonings to match.

VEGETARIAN BLACK BEAN AND HUMMUS SANDWICH WRAP

Active Time: 10 minutes
Cook Time: 15 minutes
Total Time: 25 minutes
YIELD: 2

Protein: 16 grams per serving

INGREDIENTS

- 1 (cut) onion
- 1 (cut) bell pepper
- 4 ounces sliced mushrooms
- 1/2 can of corn (rinsed and drained)
- 8 ounces roasted red bell pepper hummus (or 1 cup homemade)
- 2 large whole grain wraps
- 1/2 can of black beans (rinsed and drained)
- 1 roa roasted pepper hummus (or 1 cup homemade)
- 2 wide whole grain wraps

INSTRUCTIONS

1. Oven preheat to 450 F.
2. Sauté the onion until it becomes transparent. Add the pepper bell and simmer for 2 to 3 minutes.
3. Add the corn and mushrooms.
4. Spread the wrap onto a layer of hummus.
5. Attach the sautéed onions, rice, strips of poblano and spinach to compare.
6. Turn over into a burrito.
7. Seam side down on a baking sheet and bake for 8 to 10 minutes.

8. Serve the wrap moist, then finish with the salsa and guacamole.

POWER SALAD WITH QUINOA AND CHICKPEAS

Active Time: 15 minutes
Cook Time: 15 minutes
Total Time: 30 minutes
YIELD: 6

Protein: 12 grams per serving

INGREDIENTS

FOR THE SALAD

- 100 g quinoa - prepared according to the package instructions
- 1 jar of chickpeas - 310 g total filling weight, 265 g drained weight
- 2 carrots - peeled, coarsely grated
- 4 spring onions - finely chopped
- 50 g pistachios - chopped
- 60 g dates - chopped
- 50 g raisins
- 20 g parsley, fresh - chopped

FOR HONEY LEMON DRESSING

- 60 ml of olive oil
- 3 tablespoons of lemon juice - freshly squeezed
- 1 tbsp honey
- 1/2 teaspoon cumin - ground
- 1/2 teaspoon salt
- 1 pinch of chilli, ground - dry spice

INSTRUCTIONS

FOR THE SALAD

1. Prepare Quinoa according to the instructions and allow to cool . Whether one should wash it off hot to remove the bitter substances, the spirits argue over it. I always do it. Two more tips from me: Do not forget a good pinch of salt or use vegetable broth.
2. You can sauté the quinoa in some oil for about 1 minute (raises the nutty taste) and then add water and boil.
3. The chickpeas in a colander with water drain and rinse can.
4. The remaining or all ingredients edit and deploy. Then you mix all the ingredients together a bowl.

FOR HONEY LEMON DRESSING

5. Mix all dressing ingredients well with each other to form a homogeneous dressing.
6. Finally mix the dressing with the salad .

The longer you let the salad go, the better it tastes by the way.

VEGETARIAN MEXICAN CASSEROLE WITH BLACK BEANS

Active Time: 10 minutes

Cook Time: 15 minutes

Total Time: 25 minutes

YIELD: 8

Protein: 10 grams per serving

A Mexican casserole is sometimes called a tortilla pie, or a tortilla casserole is just a few Mexican ingredients layered in between tortillas (similar to how the lasagna is layered) and then baked in the oven.

This Mexican lacto-vegetarian casserole recipe is a great one-dish vegetarian casserole for those busy nights.

The whole family will love a simple Mexican-inspired dinner, and because this recipe takes up quite a bit, you should expect to have the leftovers.

INGREDIENTS

- 2 cups of chopped onion, fresh or frozen
- 1 1/2 cups of chopped red pepper, fresh or frozen
- 2 garlic cloves, minced
- 3/4 cup salsa
- 2 teaspoons of ground cumin
- 2 (15.8 ounce) black beans, washed
- 126-inch corn tortillas
- 2 cups of Monterey Jack and Cheddar diced
- 3 tomatoes (optional)
- 1/2 cup sliced black olives (optional)

INSTRUCTIONS

1. Oven preheat to 350 F.
2. In large skillet, mix the onion pepper, garlic, salsa, cumin and black beans and add to boil over medium heat.
3. Cook for 3 minutes, stirring frequently.
4. Arrange 6 tortillas in the bottom of a baking dish of 9 inches x 13 inches overlapping them if necessary. Place part of the mixture of beans over the tortillas and top with half the cheddar.
5. Continue the layering process with the tortillas, bean mixture and left.
6. Cover foil over the dish and bake for 15 minutes. Cut foil carefully, and serve warm.
7. Garnish with onions, olives, and sour cream.

VEGAN CROCKPOT LASAGNA WITH SPINACH AND TOFU

Active Time: 10 minutes
Cook Time: 0 minutes
Total Time: 10 minutes
Slow Cook Time:6 hrs
YIELD: 6

Protein: 12 grams per serving

You can start planning this easy vegetarian and vegan lasagna

recipe six to eight hours before dinner using just a few basic ingredients including tofu, fresh basil, frozen spinach, tomato sauce and lasagna noodles.
Using tofu helps make this lasagna recipe very low-fat and vegan, or try a vegan ricotta s substitute whether it's a grocery-bought or a homemade ricotta based on tofu.

INGREDIENTS

- 1 jar of soft (silk) tofu
- 1 tub of hard or extra firm tofu
- 1/4 cup of soy milk
- 1/2 teaspoon of garlic powder
- 2 teaspoons of lemon juice
- 3 tablespoons of fresh basil (cut)
- 1 teaspoon of salt
- 2 (10 ounces) packets of frozen spinach (thawed and patted dry)
- 4 cups of tomato sauce
- 1 (10 ounces) lasagna noodles

INSTRUCTIONS

1. Combine the silken tofu, firm or extra-firm tofu, soy milk, garlic powder, lemon juice, basil, and salt together in a food processor or blender and process until smooth.
2. Apply the mixture to the thawed spinach.
3. Put about a tomato sauce cup in the crock pot bottom, or slow cooker. So put on top of the sauce 1/3 of the lasagna noodles, and on top of the noodles 1/3 of the tofu and spinach mixture. Follow these layers, and be sure to finish with sauce on top.
4. Cook for 6 to 8 hours or until the noodles are soft in the crock pot at low heat temperature.
5. Serve with a little nutritional yeast on top, if desired. Love it!

VEGAN BLACK BEAN VEGGIE BURGERS

Active Time: 10 minutes
Cook Time: 10 minutes
Total Time: 20 minutes

Protein: 8 grams per serving

YIELD: 6

While pan-fried in a little oil, these veggie burgers cook up quickly, perfect for a quick weekday meal. But they're not yet powerful enough to throw on the bbq at the backyard. This veggie burger recipe does not include any animal products, but is not gluten-free because it uses breadcrumbs and flour.
You will not have to spend more money on frozen veggie burger patties once you get the knack of making your own veggie burgers. Plus, you control all the ingredients.

INGREDIENTS

- 1/2 onion (small cut)
- 1 (14-ounce) black beans (well drained)
- 2 slices of bread (crumbled)
- 1/2 teaspoon seasoned salt
- 1 teaspoon garlic powder
- 1 teaspoon onion powder
- 1/2 cup flour
- Dash salt (or to taste)
- Dash pepper (or to taste)
- Frying oil (split)

INSTRUCTIONS

1. Apply just enough oil to a small frying pan over medium - high heat to grease the rim. Add the onions and sauté until tender-about 3 to 5 minutes.

2. Mash the beans in a large bowl, until almost smooth.
3. Attach the sautéed onions and the crumbled potatoes, seasoned salt, garlic powder, and onion powder to the mashed black beans, and combine well.
4. Apply a few spoons of flour at a time and blend well to incorporate. Your mixture of veggie burgers will be very dense (you might want to use your hands to work the flour in well).
5.The mixture of black beans into individual patties, around 1/2 inch thick. The best way to do that is to roll a handful into a ball, and then flatten it gently.
6. Fry the black bean patties over medium-low heat in a small amount of oil until they are slightly firm and slightly brown on each side, around 3 minutes. If your pan is too dry, your bean burgers will brown too easily and will not heat up and cook in the centre, so change the heat if appropriate.
7. Assemble your veggie burgers to serve, and enjoy with all the fixings. Alternatively, eat them with a little ketchup alternatively hot sauce on a pan, and no bread. A lovely green salad can round out this into a nutritious meal.
Love it!

QUICK BREADED TOFU NUGGETS

Active Time: 45 minutes
Cook Time: 25 minutes
Total Time: 70 minutes

Protein: 6 grams per serving

YIELD: 4

Surprise your kids with a meat-free tofu nugget chicken dinner, reminiscent of the classic finger food they love to dunk in ketchup, barbecue sauce or ranch dressing.
Extra firm tofu in this dish is filled with a seasoned blend of panko breadcrumb. Then it is cooked or fried to a moist, addicting beauty just as chicken is.

As with most tofu recipes, if you first click the tofu, this one will taste best. This allows the tofu to expel additional moisture so the seasonings can be absorbed for better flavour. It also helps the tofu retain its form during the process of cooking.

INGREDIENTS

- 1 block tofu (solid or extra firm, well pressed)
- 1/3 cup of soy milk (or other non-dairy milk substitute)
- 2 tablespoons of mustard
- 1 tablespoon of nutritional yeast
- 1 teaspoon of onion powder
- 1 teaspoon of garlic powder
- 1 teaspoon of dried parsley (or Italian seasoning)
- 1/2 teaspoon of sea salt
- 1/4 teaspoon of black pepper
- 1/2 cup of panko breadcrumbs
- 3 tablespoons of high-heat vegetable oii

INSTRUCTIONS

1. Take the tofu off its package.
2. Pat the tofu block dry and put it in between two paper towel layers.
3. Place on top of the tofu a small cutting board (or flat-surface item) and a weight — like a pot or a brick.
4. Let the tofu sit for 30 minutes, when they become saturated, replace the paper towels.

Prepare For Tofu

5. Slice it into1-inch cubes or nuggets (approximately the size of a frozen chicken nugget) once your tofu is pressed.
6. Whisk the soy milk, mustard, nutritional yeast, and spices

together in a small, shallow bowl until smooth
7. Place the breadcrumbs of the panko in a separate bowl.

To fry Tofu
8. Heat the oil over medium to high heat in a frying pan.
9. Take one piece of tofu and dip it in a mixture of liquids. Then dip it gently until well covered in the breadcrumbs.
10. Remove it to the skillet and rinse.
11. Fry the bits of tofu, rotating them regularly, until all sides are golden brown.
12. Serve, and have fun!

Tofu Bake
13. Bake your tofu nuggets on a prepared baking sheet, for a low-fat alternative cooking method.
14. Preheat the oven to 350 F and bake the tofu for 25 minutes, turning once, until the brown is golden.
15. Serve and enjoy your vegetarian tofu nuggets with a ketchup, barbecue sauce or hot Sriracha sauce.

GLUTEN FREE CHOCOLATE CHIP COOKIES

Active Time: 20 minutes
Cook Time: 12 minutes
Total Time: 32 minutes
YIELD: 12

Protein: 18 grams per serving

INGREDIENTS

- 70 grams (3 and a half tablespoons) of butter
- 3/4 cup brown or blonde sugar
- 1/4 teaspoon salt

- 1 teaspoon vanilla essence
- 1/2 cup cornstarch
- 1/2 cup tapioca flour
- 1/4 cup chickpea flour
- 1 tablespoon rice flour
- 1/3 teaspoon baking soda
- 1/4 teaspoon of xanthan gum
- 1 cup chocolate chips

INSTRUCTIONS

1. Preheat the oven to 350-degree F (180 ° C).

2. In a mixer or by hand, beat the butter, sugar, and salt. It should with a creamy consistency, this takes about 5 minutes.

3. Mix the butter and add vanilla essence.

4. Add all the dry ingredients and finally the chocolate chips.

GLUTEN FREE BREAKFAST MUFFINS

Active Time: 15 minutes
Cook Time: 35 minutes
Total Time: 50 minutes

Protein: 6 grams per serving

YIELD: 8

These gluten-free muffins are healthy, satiating, easy to make and delicately sweet. This is ideal for breakfast any day. For a special breakfast, try to toast them and spread them with jam or some nut butter.

INGREDIENTS

Dry ingredients

- 2 cups of oatmeal flakes (210g), ground to flour
- 1 teaspoon baking powder
- 1/4 teaspoon of baking soda
- Pinch of salt

Liquid ingredient

- 1 cup sweet potato (265g)
- 1/2 cup of soy milk (120ml) (substitute for oat milk for a version without soy)
- 2 tablespoon maple syrup (or any other neutral flavor: agave, rice ...)
- 1 teaspoon apple cider vinegar

INSTRUCTIONS

1. First heat the oven to about 180 degrees Celsius.
2. Mix all dry ingredients in a bowl.
3. In another bowl Mix the vinegar and the milk in a bowl. Leave it for ten minutes.
4. Add the sweet potato and syrup to the bowl of milk and vinegar and combine everything well.
5. Pour the bowl with the liquid ingredients in the bowl with the dry ingredients and stir until everything is combined. Do not remove excessively or else the dough will not rise. The dough will be quite dense, and that's exactly how we want it!
6. Pour the dough into silicone molds. Place them on the lower baking sheet and bake for 35 minutes. Do not open the oven door during the baking process.

NOTES

Due to sweet potato, these muffins should be consumed in 1-2 days.

Keep in an airtight container and refrigerated.

SALAD WITH AVOCADO, CUCUMBER AND FETA

Active Time: 10 minutes
Cook Time: 5 minutes
Total Time: 15 minutes

Protein: 14 grams per serving

YIELD: 2

INGREDIENTS

- 1 avocado
- 1 cucumber
- 80 g of feta
- 10 cherry tomatoes
- 1 bunch of parsley
- The juice of 1/2 lemon
- Extra virgin olive oil
- Salt
- Salad with avocado

INSTRUCTIONS

1. Peel the avocado, cut it into cubes and sprinkle it with lemon juice.
2. Cut the cucumber into thin slices and chop the parsley coarsely.
3. In a bowl combine the avocado with the cucumber, add the chopped tomatoes and the feta into small pieces.
4. Add the chopped parsley, oil and salt.

CHICKPEA HUMMUS, AVOCADO AND BASIL

Active Time: 10 minutes
Cook Time: 15 minutes
Total Time: 25 minutes

Protein: 16 grams per serving

YIELD: 4

INGREDIENTS

- Half a ripe avocado
- 200 g of previously cooked chickpeas
- 1 lemon
- 1 clove of garlic
- About 10 g of fresh basil
- 2 teaspoons of sesame seeds
- 1/2 teaspoon of curry
- 1/2 teaspoon of paprika
- Salt to taste
-

INSTRUCTIONS

1. Ensure the avocado is washed and cut into small pieces. Cut the garlic
2. In a bowl we combine the previously cooked chickpeas (but also those in cans are fine if you haven't had time to boil them), the avocado, the chopped garlic, the basil leaves, the lemon, the sesame seeds, the curry, paprika and a pinch of salt;
3. Whisk everything with a mini immersion primer or a food processor, until the mixture has become a soft and homogeneous cream.

If it is too dry, you can add a little water.

4. Finally, if you like, you can add a dash of extra virgin olive oil and ... et voila, our delicious and healthy hummus, ready to be enjoyed

BUDDHA BOWLS
Active Time: 20 minutes
Cook Time: 20 minutes
Total Time: 40 minutes
YIELD: 2

Protein: 10 grams per serving

INGREDIENTS

- 100 g of dried chickpeas (also in an organic jar already cooked only with water) proteins
- 100 grams of bulgur carbohydrates and fiber
- 100 grams of broccoli fibers
- 1 small eggplant fiber
- 1 courgette fiber
- 1 carrot fiber
- A spoonful of tahini sauce
- 2 tablespoons of sesame oil to taste

DRESSING

- 2 tablespoons of extra virgin olive oil
- Fresh mint leaves
- The juice of ½ organic lemon
- Salt and Pepper To Taste

INSTRUCTIONS

1. Ensure the chickpeas are soaked for one night in water before boiling them for 20 minutes.
2. Cook the bulgur in twice its water weight for 15 min or as instructed in the box.
3. Wash and dry the mint and infuse it in a small bowl with extra virgin olive oil.

4. Blend half of the chickpeas cooked with 2 tablespoons of sesame oil and a tablespoon of tahini sauce and set aside.
5. Wash the broccoli and boil them, wash the courgette and cut it raw in a spiral with a spiralizer.
6. Wash the aubergine and cook it in the pan for ten minutes. salt and pepper to taste and set aside.
7. Clean the carrot with a potato peeler and make spaghetti with the spilazer.

Dressing:
8. emulsify the mint oil with the lemon, salt and pepper.

Buddha Bowls: take the bowl and arrange the vegetables, the bulgur, the legumes and the chickpea hummus in the center. Dress on the surface with the dressing.

Note
Bulgur is a food of Middle Eastern cuisine, it is a broken grain rich in fiber, a food consisting of whole wheat chopped into pieces that can be eaten as a salad (the famous Tabule), in soups, instead of rice, as a cous variant cous.

CHICKPEA FLOUR OMELETTE WITH SPINACH, BROCCOLI AND BLACK CABBAGE

Active Time: 10 minutes
Cook Time: 15 minutes
Total Time: 25 minutes
YIELD: 2

Protein: 22 grams per serving

INGREDIENTS

- 150 grams of chickpea flour
- 5 gr of whole sea salt
- 450 grams of water
- 25 grams of extra virgin olive oil
- Turmeric and pepper to taste
- Boiled broccoli, spinach and black cabbage sautéed in a pan

INSTRUCTIONS

1. In a bowl, mix flour, salt, water, oil and spices to form a smooth batter. Let the dough rest for about 3 hours.
2. Meanwhile, we prepare the vegetables (spinach, black cabbage and broccoli)
3. After the resting time of the farinata, in a non-stick frying pan with high sides, skip the vegetables, then add the dough and cover with a lid.
4. Let it cook for about 10 minutes, then, with the help of the lid, turn the omelette over and let it cook for another 5 minutes on the other side.

CHICKPEA BURGER AND TOFU

Active Time: 10 minutes
Cook Time: 15 minutes
Total Time: 25 minutes
YIELD: 4

Protein: 12 grams per serving

INGREDIENTS

- 400 g cooked chickpeas
- 275 g firm tofu
- 250 g raw mushrooms
- 40 g black olives

- Onion
- 50 g whole wheat bread
- 4 teaspoons sweet paprika
- 2 teaspoons turmeric
- 1 teaspoon ginger
- 1 teaspoon oregano
- 1 pinch of thyme
- 1 pinch of rosemary
- 1 pinch nutmeg
- 1 pinch of white pepper
- 1 pinch of black pepper
- Salt

INSTRUCTIONS

1. Chop the onion and mushrooms and sauté them with a little olive oil. Meanwhile, we drain the tofu well, undo it with our fingers and add it to the sofrito.

2. We will let it cook over medium heat until the tofu has lost all the water. In a bowl, chop the chickpeas with a fork; add the stir-fry, the sliced black olives and the spices.

3. We add the breadcrumbs little by little as we mix. If necessary, we can add more breadcrumbs until the dough is manageable and is consistent enough to form the burgers.

4. We take 150 gram dough portions and shape it. We will leave them in the pan about 5 minutes on each side or until both sides are toasted.

POTATO LEEK SOUP WITH TOFU

Active Time: 10 minutes
Cook Time: 40 minutes
Total Time: 60 minutes
YIELD: 4

Protein: 16 grams per serving

INGREDIENTS

- 150 g of potatoes
- 100 g onions
- 250 g leek
- 15 g of ginger, fresh
- 1 chili pepper, green
- 6 El oil
- 700 ml vegetable stock
- 400 ml of coconut milk
- salt
- pepper
- 2 tablespoons of lemon juice
- 250 g of broccoli
- 20 g chia seeds
- 1 tb of coriander seed

- 1 tsp sesame
- 4 spoons of pancakes
- 2 egg whites
- 250 grams of tofu

INSTRUCTIONS

1. Peel potatoes, dice roughly. Finely chop the onions. Leek, clean, wash, cut only white and light green into strips
2. Peel ginger, cut into thin strips. Halve chili lengthwise, remove seeds, cut roughly. Heat 1 tbsp. Of oil in a saucepan, sauté the prepared vegetables in a glassy sauce.
3. Fill with vegetable stock and coconut milk and bring to a boil. Season with salt, pepper and cook over medium heat for 20 minutes. Puree the soup with the cutting stick, season with lemon juice and keep warm.
4. Peel broccoli trunks. Cut broccoli with stalk into 4 pieces of 60 g each. Chia, cilantro, crushed sesame in a mortar, mix with breadcrumbs.
5. Beat the egg whites, cut the tofu into 4 slices of 60 g each, stir in the egg whites, then in crumbs. Heat 3 tablespoons of oil in the pan, fry the broccoli crispy for 4 minutes, season with salt and pepper.
6. Remove from the pan, heat remaining oil in it, roast the tofu crispy for 2-3 minutes. Drain on kitchen paper.
7. Arrange soup with broccoli and tofu in bowls, serve immediately.

CHILI SOUP WITH AVOCADO AND CORN

Active Time: 10 minutes

Cook Time: 20 minutes
Total Time: 30 minutes
YIELD: 4

Protein: 20 grams per serving

INGREDIENTS

FOR THE CORN:

- 2 fresh corncobs, the leaves and the filaments completely peeled off
- A little olive oil

FOR THE SALAD:

- 2 teaspoons extra virgin olive oil
- Juice of 1 lime, freshly squeezed
- 1/4 tsp sea salt
- Freshly ground black pepper, to taste
- 1/2 teaspoon ground cumin (cumin)
- 1 small red onion, chopped small
- 1 small red pepper, cut small
- 250 g cherry tomatoes, halved
- 1 avocado, cut small
- 1 small bunch of fresh coriander

INSTRUCTIONS

1. In a frying pan (a cast iron frying pan is recommended), heat the olive oil slightly over medium heat.
2. Next, polish the flask with a brush with a little olive oil and put it in the pan.
3. Roast covered corn cobs (approximately 3 minutes on each side, 10-12 minutes total). Then remove the flask from the pan and set it aside for cooling (approximately 10-15

minutes).
4. Once cool, use a large knife to cut the grain from the flask and place it in a bowl.
5. Add olive oil, lime juice, salt, pepper, cumin to the bowl with corn and mix well. Next, add red onion, red pepper, cherry tomatoes, avocado, fresh coriander and mix again. Enjoy

POTATO PANCAKES WITHOUT EGG

Active Time: 20 minutes
Cook Time: 10 minutes
Total Time: 30 minutes
YIELD: 2

Protein: 6 grams per serving

INGREDIENTS

- 700g potatoes
- 5 EL Flour
- 1 stk onion
- 1 TL salt
- 5 EL olive oil

INSTRUCTIONS

1. First peel for potato pancakes without egg, the onion and the potatoes and roughly grates with a grater. Mix in a bowl and salt well. Let something go.
2. Then squeeze the mixture out firmly with your hands and work in the flour. Form small buffers.
3. using a pan heat oil and fry the buffers until crispy brown on both sides for about 10 minutes.

ARUGULA SALAD WITH SWEET POTATOS

Active Time: 30 minutes
Cook Time: 15 minutes
Total Time:.45 minutes
YIELD: 4

Protein: 8 grams per serving

INGREDIENTS

- 500 gr. potatoes
- Flour
- 2 small ones white onions
- cooking oil
- vinegar
- Sugar, salt, pepper

INSTRUCTIONS

1. Boil the potatoes with while you add a pinch of salt. Heat cooking oil, add bacon cubes, sauté briefly. Then add onions and sauté briefly again.
2. First add about 1-2 l of flour and stir until the oil combines with the flour (roux forms) add about 200 ml of water, stir and bring to a boil.
3. If sauce is now too thin, add more flour if too thick. Finally, season with vinegar and sugar to create a sour-sweet sauce (add more vinegar or sugar, depending on your taste). lastly, sprinkle with pepper and a little salt, let everything boil gently.
4. Serve and enjoy

WHEAT FLOUR TORTILLAS

Active Time: 10 minutes
Cook Time: 40 minutes

Total Time: 50 minutes
YIELD: **2**

Protein: 6 grams per serving

INGREDIENTS

- 750g Flour smooth
- 300 mlwater
- 100 mloil
- 1 TL salt

INSTRUCTIONS

1. First mix all recipes until the gently rubbed or elastic dough is formed, then add water or flour to ensure proper texture. Leave to cover for at least 30 minutes.
2. Divide the dough into Twelve equal parts and spray with a small amount of flour. Warm a large coated pan and fry the fat-free tortillas from both sides for a short period of time until the dough has foamed. Leave your tortilla warm.

BUTTERNUT SQUASH SOUP

Active Time: 15 minutes
Cook Time: 40 minutes
Total Time: 55 minutes
YIELD: **2**

Protein: 10 grams per serving

INGREDIENTS

- 1stk Butternut pumpkin
- 2stk onion

- 0.5l Soup
- 3EL butter
- 1 salt and pepper
- 1 tsp nutmeg
- 1 cayenne pepper
- 0.5 cup creme fraiche

INSTRUCTIONS

1. For pumpkin soup with butternut squash , the pumpkin must be peeled and the pulp cut into cubes. Peel and finely dice the onion.
2. Braise the onion pieces in a saucepan with butter until translucent, add the pumpkin and deglaze with the soup. Simmer for about 40 minutes.
3. Then puree with the hand blender, season with salt, pepper, nutmeg and cayenne pepper. Finally, refine with creme fraiche.

VEGAN PEA SOUP

Active Time: 15 minutes
Cook Time: 20 minutes
Total Time: 35 minutes
YIELD: 4

Protein: 6 grams per serving

INGREDIENTS

- 1 stk Leek, long
- 6 stk potatoes
- 70g carrots
- 1 shot olive oil
- 2 stk stock cube

- 600g peas
- 1L water
- salt
- pepper
- Herbs (basil, parsley)

INSTRUCTIONS

1. Cut green onions, potatoes and carrots into small pieces. Prepare a large pan and add olive oil and vegetables. Let it boil for 5 minutes. Don't forget to stir many times.
2. Add water and season with soup cubes. When the water boils with vegetable fragments, peas are added, the stove is set to a weak level, and the water can boil for 1 hour 15 minutes.
3. When the peas become soft, everything is crushed until a creamy soup is made. Just season with salt, pepper, parsley and basil and serve. Good appetite!

BROCCOLI SOUP

Active Time: 20 minutes
Cook Time: 20 minutes
Total Time: 40 minutes
YIELD: 4

Protein: 14 grams per serving

INGREDIENTS

- 250g broccoli
- 1 L vegetable stock
- 1 stk Cloves of garlic (finely chopped)
- 2 EL olive oil
- 2 stk Onions (finely chopped)

- salt and pepper
- 100ml Cream

INSTRUCTIONS

1. For broccoli soup, chop broccoli, garlic and onion into small pieces and fry well in olive oil for 5 minutes.
2. Pour vegetable soup (or 3/4 water and soup cube soup) and simmer for about 20 minutes on low heat.
3. Finally, mix it briefly with a hand blender and season with salt and pepper.

It can be refined by adding cream.

LENTIL MUSHROOM MEATLESS PASTA (BOLOGNESE)

Active Time: 10 minutes
Cook Time: 15 minutes
Total Time: 25 minutes
YIELD: 4

Protein: 12.5 grams per serving

INGREDIENTS

- 2 tablespoons of olive oil (OF: 1/4 cup / 60 ml quinococcus)
- 1 large yellow onion, finely chopped
- 2 Portobello mushrooms or 1 10 oz (283 g) package of cremini mushrooms, trimmed and minced
- 2 tablespoons of tomato paste
- 3 garlic, chopped
- 1 teaspoon oregano
- 2 1/2 cup (600 ml) of water
- 1 cup brown lentils (200 g)
- Puree or diced 28 oz (794 g) tomatoes with basil (diced juice)

- 1 tablespoon balsamic vinegar
- Pasta
- Salt and black pepper
- chopped basil

INSTRUCTIONS

1. Place a large stock pot on medium heat. Add oil. When the oil has warmed up (or the soup has started to boil), add the onions and mushrooms. Cover and cook for about 5 minutes until both are soft. Add tomato paste, garlic and oregano, cook for 2 minutes and constantly stir.

2. Stir the water and lentils. Bring to a boil, lower to medium heat and cook for 5 minutes. Add the tomatoes (juice if diced) and vinegar. Cover, reduce heat and cook for about 30 minutes until lentils are soft.

3. Cook the pasta according to the instructions on the package.

4. Remove the sauce from the fire and season with salt and pepper. Decorate with basil and serve over pasta.

Early: Use cooked lentils. It is available in cans or in a sealed package in a refrigerated vegetable cooler. If you take this route, omit the recipe water, cook the sauce on medium heat for about 20 minutes, and finally stir and heat the lentils.

ALMOND BUTTER TOFU STIR-FRY

Active Time: 15 minutes
Cook Time: 50 minutes
Total Time: 1 hour 5minutes
YIELD: 2

Protein: 12 grams per serving

INGREDIENTS

Tofu

- 1 extra 12 oz package extra farm tofu

Marinade

- 2 tablespoons sesame oil (divided)
- 4 tablespoons of low salt pool (or soy sauce if not GF)
- 3 tablespoons maple syrup
- 2 tablespoons almond butter (or sub peanut butter)
- 2 tablespoons lime juice
- 1-2 teaspoon pepper garlic sauce

Vegetables

- 1 pound of green beans (trimmed)
- 2-3 small spicy peppers (I used cherry bombs-use peppers to reduce heat)

INSTRUCTIONS

1. Preheat oven to 400 degrees F (204 C) and spread parchment on baking sheet. Also wrap the tofu in a clean, absorbent towel and place a heavy object on top, such as a cast iron skillet, to push out excess moisture.
2. Once the oven is preheated, uncook the tofu and cut into small cubes. Make a flat layer on a lined baking sheet and bake for 25-30 minutes or plump and dry until the edges are slightly crisp (see photo). This step makes the tofu crispy. The longer it is baked, the harder and crisp it becomes, so adjust the cooking time accordingly.

3. Meanwhile, add half a sesame oil (1 tablespoon written as original recipe / adjust if changing batch size), puddle, maple syrup, almond butter, lime juice, chilli garlic sauce / red in a small mixing bowl Masu pepper flakes / Thai pepper. Mix and whisk. Then adjust the taste and taste as needed, adding creamy / nut almond butter, salty puddles, sour lime juice, or hot chili garlic sauce. Set aside.

4. If you want to serve with rice, prepare at this point (see note). Add the roasted tofu to the almond butter Tama resource and marinade for 5 minutes with occasional stirring. The longer the marinating time, the stronger the flavor, but it turns out that 5 to 10 minutes is enough.
5. Heat a large skillet over medium heat. When warm, add the tofu and leave most of the marinade (this is added for the flavor of the vegetables).
6. Cook for about 5 minutes, stirring occasionally, until all sides turn brown and slightly caramel. Remove from bread and set aside.
7. In a frying pan, put the remaining sesame oil (1 tablespoon as the original recipe is written // adjust if changing batch size), 2-3 beans of green beans and peppers (30-45 ml // original recipe is written If you want to change the batch size of the marinade to adjust // the amount as it is).
8. Steam for about 4-5 minutes or until the green beans are soft. Then remove the lid, raise the heat to medium heat and add the remaining marinade and tofu. Cook for another 1-2 minutes with frequent agitation. Then remove from heat.

9. Serve as is or on cooked or cauliflower rice. For additional heat, add chili garlic sauce or sriracha. Keep the leftovers in the refrigerator for up to 3 days. Reheat on stove or microwave until hot.

ROMESCO SOUP WITH SMASHED CHICKPEAS

Active Time: 25 minutes
Cook Time: 5 minutes
Total Time: 30minutes
YIELD: 4

Protein: 10 grams per serving

INGREDIENTS

Soup

- 2 large red peppers (with skin // with stem)
- 1 cup of raw almonds
- 4 garlic crusts (with skin)
- 1 28 oz diced tomatoes (slightly drained // like San Marzano)
- 4 cups of vegetable soup (DIY or commercially available)
- 1 1/2 tablespoon red wine vinegar (to reduce acidity and / or sub-apple cider vinegar)
- 3/4 teaspoon smoked paprika (for more taste)
- 1/2 teaspoon of sea salt and black pepper
- 1 tablespoon maple syrup or coconut sugar (or taste stevia-just a little)
- Harissa paste 1-2 teaspoon (optional 1/4 teaspoon red pepper flakes more or less depending on preference)
- 1 15 oz chickpeas (rinse)

Optional offer

- Vegan parmesan cheese
- Whole grain bread or simple vegan roll
- Fresh herbs (parsley or coriander)

- Pine nut

INSTRUCTIONS

1. Preheat the oven to 350 degrees Fahrenheit (176 C) and place a red pepper with still whole stems on one side of a clean baking sheet. On the other end, place almonds and garlic (still on the skin). If you need to create a larger batch, use more tops as needed.

2. Place the baking sheet in the oven and roast the almonds for 10 to 12 minutes or until slightly cracked and golden. Next, remove the almonds from the pot and save them. Bake the garlic for another 5-8 minutes. Then remove and set aside.
3. Heat the peppers to 475 degrees F (246 C) with the peppers on the baking sheet. Roast the red pepper until the skin is foamy and mostly black, turn halfway upside down and burn both sides (about 10 minutes).
4. Once cooked, wrap the red pepper in foil and steam for 2-3 minutes. Next, peel the skin, seeds and core. Also remove the roasted garlic crust.
5. Add peeled pepper, almonds, garlic, diced tomatoes, vinegar, paprika, sea salt, hu pepper, maple syrup, or coconut sugar, and (optional) harissa or hupper flakes to the high speed blender . Scrape the sides as necessary until smooth. Taste and adjust the seasonings to your liking, adding harissa or pepper flakes for heat, salt for salty, maple syrup or coconut sugar for acidity, paprika for smokyness.

6. Put the soup in a large pan and add the vegetable soup and chickpeas. Cook over medium heat. Afterwards, lower the heat and simmer for 10-15 minutes, stirring occasionally.
7. Serve as is or with pine nuts, fresh herbs, vegan parmesan cheese, or your favorite bread or roll.

The leftovers are well covered in the refrigerator for 3-4 days, but are best when fresh.

BLISSED-OUT THAI SALAD WITH PEANUT TEMPEH

Active Time: 25 minutes
Cook Time: 5 minutes
Total Time: 30minutes
YIELD: 4

Protein: 10 grams per serving

INGREDIENTS

Salad

- 6 oz vermicelli noodles (I like brown rice noodles)
- 2 medium-sized carrots "ribbon-shaped" with vegetable peeler or spiralizer
- 2 green onions (finely chopped)
- 1/4 cup chopped coriander
- 2-3 tablespoons of minced mint
- 1 cup spinach (chopped)
- 1 cup sliced red cabbage
- 1 medium red pepper (sliced)
- 1 batch of peanut tempe marinade (optional)

Dressing

- 1/3 cup salty creamy peanut butter, almond butter or sun butter
- 3 tablespoons of gluten free tamari (or soy sauce if not GF)
- 3 tablespoons maple syrup
- 1 tsp chili garlic sauce
- 1 medium lime, juice (3 tablespoons or 45 ml)

- 1/4 cup water (thin)

INSTRUCTIONS

1. Cook, rinse, drain and cool rice noodles
2. In a large serving bowl, add the cooked and cooled noodles, carrots, green onions, coriander, mint, spinach, cabbage and red peppers and mix gently. Set aside.
3. Add peanut butter, pool, maple syrup, chili sauce (or chili or red pepper) and lime juice to a small mixing bowl, whisk and mix to make the dressing. Then add warm water in small portions until you have a thick, pourable sauce.
4. Taste and adjust seasonings as needed. Add maple syrup for sweetness, chili sauce (chili or red pepper) for heat, lime juice for sourness, and puddles for salty. Set aside.
5. Add half of Tempe (optional) and half of sauce to salad and toss. Then top with the remaining tempe and sauce. Please put it out immediately. The leftovers can be stored in the refrigerator for 4-5 days, but are best when fresh. If you make it in advance, I think it's better to remove the salad and store tempe separately.

SMOKY TEMPEH BURRITO BOWLS

Active Time: 1hour 15 minutes
Cook Time: 30 minutes
Total Time: 1 hour 45 minutes
YIELD: 3

Protein: 14 grams per serving

INGREDIENTS

Rice + beans

- 1 cup of raw cup + cooking water

- 1 15 oz canned black beans (add salt if saltless)
- 1/2 teaspoon cumin powder

Tempe

- 10 oz tempe (GF * // guaranteed gluten free for cubes)
- 1 tablespoon olive or avocado oil

Marinade

- 1 tablespoon olive or avocado oil
- 1/2 large white onion (dice)
- 2 pieces of garlic, chopped (1 tablespoon with 2 pieces)
- 1 15 oz canned tomato sauce *
- 1 tipotle of advo sauce (canned // plus 1 tablespoon sauce // adjusted to your favorite spice)

Optional offer serving

- Fresh coriander, chopped
- Red cabbage, sliced
- Hot sauce

INSTRUCTIONS

1. If you want to serve with rice, use this method from Saveur. It will take 45 minutes, so start now and start the service.
2. Next, add 1 inch of water to a large pot and stew to create a tempe of steam. Next, insert the steamer basket and cover with tempe (still cut into whole or large chunks). Cover and steam for 15 minutes. This softens the texture slightly, and most importantly, brings out some bitterness. After steaming, cube and save.
3. Heat a medium cast iron or metal pan over medium heat to make the sauce. When hot, add the oil and onion. Cook with frequent stirring until soft and slightly brown-3 minutes. Then add the garlic and cook for another 1-2 minutes.

4. Add tomato sauce, tipo pepper and adobo sauce and stir. Heat until lather, reduce heat and simmer for 3-4 minutes.
5. Transfer the sauce to a blender for a high blend, completely smooth sauce. For chunky sauces, pulsate and leave the texture (in my case it should be smooth).
6. Taste and adjust seasonings as needed, add a little salt to increase flavor, and add advo sauce to heat.
7. Return the sauce to the pan and heat over low heat with occasional stirring to thicken the sauce and deepen the flavor. Then add the black beans to a small pot and heat over medium heat. If foamy, reduce heat, add a pinch of cumin and sea salt, stir and lower to low / low heat (to warm up to serving). For the texture of the refried bean, mash it under a wooden spoon until it is thick and pasty (I left the whole thing).
8. Heat another large frying pan over medium heat. Once warm, add oil and cubic (steamed) tempe, add crisp and brown to the whole-about 6-8 minutes total. Next, add the red sauce and stir gently to coat.
9. Cover the flavor with a lid for 2-3 minutes, dissolve the flavor, remove the lid and continue baking to very low temperatures.
10. To serve, divide rice, beans, tempe, and vegetables into 2-3 serving bowls. Decorate with lime and fresh coriander (optional). Keep the leftovers covered in the refrigerator for up to 3 days.

NOURISHING CURRIED LENTIL & SWEET POTATO BOWL

Active Time: 10 minutes
Cook Time: 20 minutes
Total Time: 30 minutes
YIELD: 4

Protein: 10 grams per serving

INGREDIENTS

Lentil

- 1 batch of coconut curry golden lentils

Potato

- 1 large sweet potato (round or small wedges // skin // organic if possible)
- 2 tablespoons of coconut or avocado oil (see note for oil-free *)
- 1/4 teaspoon sea salt

Cauliflower rice

- 1 head cauliflower (grated "rice" and / or semi-cooked white or brown rice)
- 1 tbsp oil or water
- 1 pinch sea salt
- 1/2 tsp curry powder (optional)

Kale

- 1 bunch of organic kale or collard green (chopped // other green // or coconut curry green)

Optional offer for serving

- 1 batch coriander chutney
- Sliced red cabbage
- Fresh coriander
- Comb lime

INSTRUCTIONS

1. Make coconut curry golden lentils.
2. Preheat oven to 375 degrees F (190 C) and place parchment on baking sheet.

Add sweet potato, oil *, salt and toss and mix. Bake for 20-25 minutes or until soft and slightly brown on the edges.
3. In the meantime, heat the large skillet over medium heat to prepare the cauliflower rice. When hot, add oil or water, cauliflower rice, salt and curry powder. Mix.
4. Reduce heat, fry for 3-5 minutes, steam and stir occasionally. Adjust the taste as needed. Set aside.
5. Next, heat the frying pan or pan over high heat and add 1/2 inch of water to prepare the kale. Bring to a boil. Next, put the steamer basket on top. Add kale and cover. Steam for 2-3 minutes or until wilted and bright green. Remove from the pan and save.
6. Finally, prepare the remaining serving items such as chutney, sliced cabbage and coriander (all optional).
7. Enjoy sweet potatoes, curry lentils, cauliflower rice, kale and other items in a bowl.
8. Store the remaining ingredients in the refrigerator for 3-4 days.

VEGAN MUSHROOM BOLOGNESE
Active Time: 20 minutes
Cook Time: 40 minutes
Total Time: 60 minutes

Protein: 11 grams per serving

YIELD: 4

INGREDIENTS

- Half onion,
- 1 small carrot coarsely chopped (1/2 cup)
- 1 coarsely chopped celery stem (1/3 cup)
- 227 g Cremini or King Oyster mushrooms, coarsely chopped

- 3 tablespoons olive oil, coarsely chopped
- 1/4 teaspoon salt
- 1 540 mL red kidney beans
- 3 garlics, chopped
- 2 tablespoons tomato paste
- 1/2 teaspoon smoked paprika
- 1/8 teaspoon of cinnamon
- 1/4 cup of dry red wine
- 1 cup vegetable soup
- 1 398 mL diced tomato
- 5 thyme twig
- Fett Cheer Rich Anoodle

INSTRUCTIONS

1. Mix cabbage, carrots and celery in a food processor. Pulse, scraping down the side as desired, until 1/4-in
2. Switch to a wide tub. Pulse the mushrooms, in batches, to 1/2-in. Parts, then move to the vegetable pot.
3. Place a pot over low pressure. Add 2 tablespoons of butter, then vegetables and salt. Heat, stirring regularly, until the vegetable mixture tends to be hot, 9 to 10 min
4. DRAIN beans in a cup, conserve the liquid. Whirl the beans in the food processor before purée. Add 2 to 3 tbsp of the stored liquid until the mixture is smooth and 1 1/2 cups thick.
5. Add the remaining 2 tsp of butter, garlic, tomato paste, paprika and cinnamon to the vegetables. Cook, stirring frequently, until the mixture begins to adhere to the pan, around 2 min.
6. Attach the wine and clean some browned pieces with a wooden spoon. Mix the bean purée, the water, the tomatoes and the thyme sprigs.
7. Bring to a boil, simmer over medium-low heat, stirring

periodically, until warm, around 18 to 20 min. Drop the thyme sprigs before eating.
8. Serve with spaghetti or polenta.

CRISPY TOFU STIR FRY WITH PEANUT SAUCE

Active Time: 15 minutes
Cook Time: 15 minutes
Total Time: 30 minutes

Protein: 26 grams per serving

YIELD: 4

INGREDIENTS

- 1 350 g super hard tofu cut into 1/4 inch thick triangles
- 2 tsp cornstarch
- 1/2 teaspoon
- 1/2 teaspoon pepper
- 1 tbsp canola oil, split
- 1113g shii, stem and half
- 4 cups of green beans, trimmed in half
- Two 100g ramen
- 2 tsp sesame oil
- 2 sliced green onions
- 1/3 cup of roasted salted peanuts, roughly chopped
- Source
- 1/3 cup smooth natural peanut butter
- 2 1/2 tbsp lime juice
- 5 tsp low sodium soy sauce
- 4 tsp honey
- 2 cups of chili sauce such as Sambal Oelec

INSTRUCTIONS

1. Take a large pot of water to a boil.

Sauce: Whisk peanut butter in a small dish, with lime juice, soy sauce, sugar, chili paste and 2/3 cup hot tea.

2. Pat fresh tofu with cooking towel. Toss until well mixed with cornstarch, salt, and pepper.
3. Heat medium - high over an extra-large non-stick frying pan.
4. Add 1 tsp of canola oil, and then half the tofu. Cook, flipping halfway through, 4 to 5 min, until golden brown, Switch into a platform. Repeat with 1 tsp of canola oil, and tofu left. Move to similar tray.
5. Remove 1 tsp of canola oil left, then mushrooms. Stir-fry before the mushrooms begin browning, around 2 min. Remove beans and cook for 3 to 4 min, until tender-crisp. Take off fire.
6. Toss the mixture of tofu and peanut butter until well powdered.
7. Cook the noodles in a pot of boiling water, following the instructions of the packet but omitting the seasoning mixture, 2 to 3 min until tender. Return to the pot and rinse, then toss with the sesame oil.
8. Divide the noodles into four bowls and finish with stir-fry tofu, green onions and peanuts. Serve straightaway.

CRISPY SPICY TOFU NOODLE BOWL

Active Time: 10 minutes
Cook Time: 15 minutes
Total Time: 25 minutes

Protein: 24 grams per serving

YIELD: 4

INGREDIENTS

- 180 g buckwheat, (about 2 1-inch bundles)
- 350 g tofu, extra firm, cut to 1/2 inch. Cube
- Pepper
- 3 tablespoons of corn starch
- 2 tablespoons sesame oil
- 2 tablespoons soy sauce, low sodium
- 5 tsp honey
- 1 tablespoon of gochujang
- 1/2 cup green soybeans, thawed
- 3 mini cucumbers, sliced
- 6 radishes, sliced
- 2 green onions, sliced

INSTRUCTIONS

1. Cook noodles in a big pot of boiling water, following the instructions of the packet, but omitting salt, 4 min. until tender. Drain the noodles, then rinse in cool broth.

2. Pat tofu dry with towels made from cotton. Spray with cinnamon, then toss in a small bowl of cornstarch. Heat media-high over a large non-stick frying pan, Add 1 tbsp of sesame oil, and add some tofu. Cook, sometimes turning the cubes until crispy and golden-colored, 5 to 7 min. Move to a platter filled with paper towels.

3. Stir the vinegar in a large bowl with soy sauce, butter, gochujang and remaining sesame oil. Drain noodles and shake the mixture with the vinegar. For mix, add edamame, cucumbers, radishes, green onions and tofu.

4. Divide noodles and mixtures of tofu into 4 cups.

SHEET PAN SESAME TOFU WITH ROASTED VEGETABLES

Active Time: 20 minutes
Cook Time: 25 minutes
Total Time: 45 minutes

Protein: 16 grams per serving

YIELD: 4

INGREDIENTS

- 1/3 cup rice vinegar
- 2 1/2 tablespoon brown sugar
- 2 1/2 tbsp reduced salt soy sauce
- 1 1/2 tablespoon sesame oil
- 2 garlic pieces, chopped
- 1 tablespoon of grated raw inger
- 1 350-g pkg firm tofu
- 2 tbsp vegetable oil
- One 400 g bundle carrot, 4 splits
- Two 170g Pack King Oyster Mushrooms Sliced
- 2 cups of green beans
- 1 tbsp chili garlic sauce, (optional)

INSTRUCTIONS

1. Position racks in upper and lower thirds of oven. Up to 400f. Whisk a casserole dish of vinegar, butter, corn, salt, garlic and ginger.
2. For drizzling save 1/4 cup of the mixture. Remove tofu, and marinate for 15 min, turning periodically. Cut, and break into 2 rimmed baking sheets.

3. Whisk in marinade vegetable oil. Attach carrots and mushrooms then turn over blanket. Divide between sheets to crust, thenroast for 10 min. Stir in the beans on both sides, then turn to top and bottom sides and simmer until the beans are tender-crisp, 10 min.
4. Drizzle vegetables with 1/4 cup marinade reserved, tossing to cover. Until serving, spoon chilli-garlic sauce over tofu.

VEGETARIAN HAGGIS COTTAGE PIE

Active Time: 15 minutes
Cook Time: 25 minutes
Total Time: 40 minutes

Protein: 17 grams per serving

YIELD: 4

INGREDIENTS

- 2 peeled and cut Yukon gold potatoes (about 850g)
- 1 227-g Pack Cremini Mushroom
- 1 onion, coarsely chopped
- 1 carrot, peeled and coarsely chopped
- 1/4 cup butter, split
- 1 540 mL canned lentils, drain, rinse
- 1/2 cup large flake oats
- 2 tablespoons soy sauce
- 1 tbsp tomato paste
- 3/4 teaspoon nutmeg
- 1/2 teaspoon pepper
- 1 cup frozen green peas
- 1/4 teaspoon salt

INSTRUCTIONS

1. Combine the potatoes in a small pot with enough water to cover. Bring to a boil, and simmer for 10 to 12 min until tender. Drain well, and put potatoes back to the pot.
2. Pulse the mushrooms until finely chopped in a food processor. Fall into a tub. Add carrot and onion to food processor, pulse until finely chopped.
3. Melt 1 tbsp of butter over medium-high in a large frying pan which is suitable for the oven. Remove the mushrooms and cook until there is almost no liquid left, 6 to 8 min.
4. Attach 1 tbsp of butter, then blend with the onion. Cook, stirring constantly until cooled, for 3 to 4 min. Add lentils, peas, 1 1/2 cups of tea, soy sauce, tomato paste, nutmeg and pepper. Bring to a boil then rising to medium heat.
5. Cook, stirring regularly, for 10 to 12 minutes, until the oats are soft and the mixture is still saucy. Place the peas in the upper third of the oven, then preheat the broiler, about 2 min.
6. Mash the potatoes until smooth with remaining 2 tbsp butter and salt. Using potato mixture to scatter over lentil mixture, Broil for 2 to 3 minutes before golden brown.

HERB FALAFELS WITH SMASHED CUCUMBER SALAD

Active Time: 20 minutes
Cook Time: 20 minutes
Total Time: 40 minutes

Protein: 11 **grams per serving**

YIELD: 4

INGREDIENTS

- 6 mini cucumbers
- 1 1/2 teaspoon salt
- 1 Add chickpea to 540 mL without salt, drain, and rinse.
- 1 egg beaten
- 1 onion, finely chopped
- 1 1/2 cup chopped parsley
- 1 cup chopped dill
- 1/4 cup general purpose flour
- 1 1/2 teaspoon of garlic powder
- 1 teaspoon cumin
- 1 teaspoon coriander
- 1/2 teaspoon baking powder
- 3 1/2 teaspoon olive oil
- 2 tablespoons white wine vinegar
- 1 teaspoon of Dijon mustard
- 1/4 teaspoon za'atar, split
- 4 cups baby spinach
- 1/4 cup crushed feta cheese

INSTRUCTIONS

1. Smash the cucumbers with a rolling pin or a small pot at the rim, then break into 1-in. Parts.
2. Place in a strainer and use 1/2 tsp salt to shake. Let stand to wash out some moisture, about 30 min. Pound chickpeas in a large bowl with a potato masher until crumbly.
3. Add the potato, onion, spices, rice, seasonings, baking powder and 1 tsp of salt until well mixed.
4. Scoop the mixture into patties, each about 1/2 in, with a 1/4 cup measure and form. Solid. Set aside on a baking dish. Heat a large frying pan over hot. (You will have about 12 patties.)
5. Add 2 tbsp of oil to plate, and half of the patties. Fry, 4 to 5 min.

per hand, before golden. Match for extra patties.
6. In a wide tub, whisk the remaining 1 1/2 tbsp of oil with vinegar, dijon and 1/8 tsp za'atar. Cast on cucumbers. Stir the spinach into the cucumbers before separating into 4 plates.
7. Sprinkle with feta and falafels on top. Sprinkle overtop with remaining 1/8 tsp of za'atar.

TOFU KEDGEREE

Active Time: 10 minutes
Cook Time: 20 minutes
Total Time: 30 minutes
Protein: 16 grams per serving

YIELD: 4

INGREDIENTS

- 2 tablespoons canola oil
- 1 finely chopped onion
- 2 garlic pieces, chopped
- 2 1/2 tsp curry powder
- 1 cup basmati rice
- 1 3/4 cup vegetable soup
- 1/2 cup sultana raisin
- 1/2 teaspoon salt
- 3 cups cauliflower florets
- 1 210 g smoked tofu, cut to 1/2 inch. strip
- 4 cups of coarsely chopped baby spinach
- 2 tablespoons chopped cilanto

INSTRUCTIONS

1. Position rack in the middle of the oven, then 400f preheat.

Attach foil to a baking dish.
2. Heat 1 tbsp of oil in a large over medium frying pan. Attach the onion, garlic, and curry powder with 2 tsp. Cook for 3 to 4 min, until the onion is tender. Stir the rice back.
3. Stir in milk, raisins and 1/4 tsp of salt. Carry to simmer. Reduce heat to medium-low and simmer, coated with 1/2 tsp curry powder and 1/4 tsp salt on prepared surface, until rice is only tender and liquid is absorbed, 12 to 15 min.
4. Roast for 10 minutes, then add tofu to the baking sheet and proceed to roast until tender-crisp, about 15 min. Remove rice from heat and mix in spinach until wilted.
5. Move to bowl. Finish kedgeree with cauliflower, cilantro and tofu.

GRILLED SATAY TOFU SKEWERS

Active Time: 30 minutes
Cook Time: 60 minutes
Total Time: 90 minutes

Protein: 15 grams per serving

YIELD: 4

INGREDIENTS

- 1 350g super hard tofu
- 1 Coconut milk in 165 mL can
- 2 tbsp yellow curry paste
- 1 tablespoon brown sugar
- 1 tablespoon smooth natural peanut butter
- 2 tsp soy sauce

INSTRUCTIONS

1. Soak 8 wooden skewers in hot water for 20 minutes. Poke holes with a skewer all over tofu. Pat dry and cut into 3/4-in paper towels. Cubicles. In a small dish, whisk the coconut milk, curry paste, brown sugar, peanut butter and soy sauce.
2. Attach tofu to cover, and throw. Set aside to marinate to medium for 1 hour. Preheat barbecue.
3. Shake the tofu off extra marinade and back into the tub. Divide the marinated tofu into skewers and cord.
4. Marinate the scrape into a small saucepan and put over medium-high. Heat, stirring regularly, until mixture is halved, 5 to 6 min. Deposit back.
5.Grill oil. Grill skewers, lid closed, turning every 1 to 2 minutes before markings on the grill surface. Brush satay sauce. Serve the salad and rice with thai basil and cilantro.

TUSCAN WHITE BEAN AND TOMATO PASTA

Active Time: 15 minutes
Cook Time: 10 minutes
Total Time: 25 minutes

Protein: 11 grams per serving
YIELD: 6

INGREDIENTS

- 250 g of whole wheat linguine pasta
- 1/3 cup of olive oil
- 1 1/2 cup breadcrumbs
- 1 teaspoon salt
- 3/4 cup chopped parsley

- 1 garlic, chopped
- 1 onion, chopped
- 1/2 teaspoon pepper
- 3 cups of cherry tomatoes in half
- 1 540-mL canned kidney beans, drain, rinse

INSTRUCTIONS

1. Carry a salted bowl of water to a boil. Cook pasta as instructed in the box, reserving 1 cup of pasta water.
2. Heat 1/4 cup oil in a large over medium frying pan. Add the bread crumbs and 1/2 tsp salt and fry, stirring constantly for about 4 minutes until golden.
3. Incorporate parsley and garlic, then move to a pot, scrap pan good.

Over medium heat remaining 2 tbsp of oil in the same tub. Add onion, remaining 1/2 tsp salt and pepper and simmer for around 6 minutes until softened.

4. Remove tomatoes and cook until tender, add rice, beans and rice water for around 8 min.
5. Add, tossing until well coated. Divide between bowls, scatter generously with crumbs of bread.

SUPERFOOD SANDWICH

Active Time: 10 minutes
Cook Time: 5 minutes
Total Time: 15 minutes

Protein: 10 grams per serving

YIELD: 1

INGREDIENTS

- 2 coarse brown breads, the following recipe link
- Edamame creamy spread, below recipe link
- Boston lettuce
- Pickled red onion, recipe link below
- Raw beetroot
- Sliced raw radish
- Sliced avocado
- Buffalo mozzarella cheese
- Subrahummus

INSTRUCTIONS

Layer sliced coarse brown bread with creamy edamame spread, lettuce, pickled red onion, radish, radish, avocado, mozzarella, sprouts and hummus.

MOCHA TOFU MOUSSE

Active Time: 5 minutes
Cook Time: 3 hours
Total Time: 3 hours 5 minutes

Protein: 7 grams per serving

YIELD: 4

INGREDIENTS

- 3/4 cup milk chocolate chips
- Silky tofu
- 2 tablespoons sugar-free cocoa powder

- 1/2 teaspoon instant coffee granules
- 1/2 teaspoon vanilla
- Raspberry, optional

INSTRUCTIONS

1. Microwave chocolate chips up to molten in a small bowl at warm, mixing halfway through, 1 to 2 min. Stir until completely cooled.
2. Whirl tofu coated with sugar, instant coffee and cinnamon until smooth. Scrape and whirl in hot chocolate until smooth and mixed.
3. Scrape pudding into 4 cups for dessert. Cover and refrigerate for at least 3 hours or overnight, until chilled and slightly solid. When needed serve with fresh raspberries.

BLACK RICE AND EDAMAME SALAD

Active Time: 15 minutes
Cook Time: 20 minutes
Total Time: 35 minutes

Protein: 6 grams per serving

YIELD: 3

INGREDIENTS

- Edamame with cupped shell, thawed
- 8 shiitake mushrooms, sliced, about 1/2 cup
- 1/8 teaspoon of kosher salt
- 1 cup black rice, rinse well
- 2 tablespoons of reduced salt soy sauce
- 1 tablespoon rice vinegar
- 1 1/2 teaspoon honey or agave syrup

- 3/4 teaspoon of sesame oil
- 1/4 cup sliced green onion
- 1/4 cup coarsely chopped coriander

INSTRUCTIONS

1. Boil water in a large pot for 3 1/2 cups. Add mushrooms and edamame. Cook for 1 min, then scrape with a sieve or strainer. Clean under cool running spray, edamame and mushrooms, and wash properly.
2. Add salt and rice to the same frying pan. Reduce heat to medium-low, as water returns to boil. Simmer, sealed, about 20 min, until rice is only tender. Rinse rice, until crisp, under cold running water. Drain fine.
3. Whisk the soy in a large bowl with sugar, honey and sesame oil. Add edamame, mushrooms, beans, cilantro and green onions. Stir until well coated.

ONE-PAN MUSHROOM GRATIN WITH WHITE BEANS

Active Time: 15 minutes
Cook Time: 30 minutes
Total Time: 45 minutes

Protein: 24 grams per serving

YIELD: 4

INGREDIENTS

- 3 tablespoons olive oil
- 2 227-g pkg cremini mushrooms, quartered (6 cups)
- 1 onion, chopped
- 2 garlic pieces, chopped

- 1/4 teaspoon salt
- 1/4 teaspoon pepper
- 1 1/4 cup unsalted vegetable soup
- 3 cups of canned white beans, drain, rinse (approx. 11/2 cans)
- 4 fried rice
- 1/2 cup panko
- Finely grated Parmesan 1/2 cup (optional)
- 2 tablespoons chopped parsley

INSTRUCTIONS

1. Preheat to 425f.
2. Heat 2 tbsp of oil over medium - high, in a large oven-safe frying pan. Remove mushrooms, and cook until browning, 9 min. Attach onion, garlic, salt and pepper and minimize to mild.
3. Cook for 5 min, until softened. Remove broth and stir up brown pieces from the bottom of the tub. Stir in beans and put to a boil. Reduce to medium-low, boil for about 8 minutes.
4. In a small pot, mix in swiss chard and cook until wilted, 2 min. Add panko, parmesan, parsley and 1 tbsp remaining oil. Sprinkle the paste over the beans.
5. Bake for 8 to 10 minutes, until top is white.

HUEVOS RANCHEROS

Active Time: 10 minutes
Cook Time: 10 minutes
Total Time: 20 minutes

Protein: 13 grams per serving

YIELD: 4

INGREDIENTS

- 1 tbsp canola oil, split
- 1 garlic, chopped
- 1/2 teaspoon cumin
- 1 cup of canned black beans, drain, rinse
- 1/2 cup of water
- 1 tablespoon lime juice
- 4 eggs
- 4 soft corn or flour tortillas
- 1/3 cup of crushed feta cheese

INSTRUCTIONS

1. Heat over liquid-high medium saucepan. Add 1 tsp of butter, then substitute the cumin and garlic. Stir constantly, 1 min, until fragrant. Season with beans and water
2. Start cooking until the beans are soft and drink much of the oil, 6 to 7 min. Apply lime juice. Mash gently with a potato masher.
3. Heat the medium in a large non-stick oven. Remove the remaining 2 tsp of oil and smash the eggs into the saucepan.
4. Cook, wrapped, until eggs are set, but yolks are still runny, 2 to 3 min. Put on a plate a tortilla.
5. Fill with rice, and then with egg and feta.

LEMON BEAN DIP

Active Time: 10 minutes
Cook Time: 10 minutes
Total Time: 20 minutes

Protein: 6 grams per serving

YIELD: 4

INGREDIENTS

- 1 540-mL canned sponge beans, drain, rinse
- 2 garlic pieces, chopped
- 1 tablespoon lemon peel
- 3 tablespoons of lemon juice
- 5 tablespoons olive oil
- 2 tablespoons of parsley, plus garnish (optional)

INSTRUCTIONS

1. Turn the beans, garlic, skin and juice with a food processor until smooth.
2. Run the motor and add 4 tbsp oil and parsley.
3. Scrape into a bowl and add the remaining 1 tbsp oil and parsley. Serve with Kurdite, Crostini and crackers.
4. Store refrigerated for 3 days

INDIAN CHICKPEA PIZZA WITH LIME RAITA

Active Time: 20 minutes
Cook Time: 20 minutes
Total Time: 40 minutes

Protein: 16 grams per serving

YIELD: 4
INGREDIENTS

- 1 tablespoon of canola oil
- 1 onion, finely chopped
- 1 tablespoon ginger
- 1 red pepper diced

- 1 zucchini, diced
- 1 tablespoon of tandoori curry paste
- 1/4 cup and 1 tbsp water
- 1 cup chickpea, drain, rinse
- 1/4 teaspoon salt
- Nan bread 4 pieces
- 1/2 cup of grated mozzarella cheese
- 1/3 cup 2% yogurt
- 1 tablespoon lime juice
- 1/4 cup chopped coriander

INSTRUCTIONS

1. Preheat oven to 400F. Heat oil over medium in a large frying saucepan. For turn, add the cabbage, ginger, red pepper and zucchini.
2. Cook for around 5 min, until vegetables are tender. Attach the curry paste with tandoori, 1/4 cup sugar, chickpeas and butter. Cook another 2 min. Mash the chickpeas softly in a saucepan.
3. Place Naan Place on baking sheet. Divide vegetable blend between breads. Add mozzarella to scatter.
4. Bake in the middle of the oven before the cheese melts. STIR Stir yogurt in a small bowl of lime juice and 1 tbsp of water.
5. Brush over moist pizzas, then scatter with coriander.

HALLOUMI AND SWEET POTATO SKEWERS WITH LENTIL SALAD

Active Time: 20 minutes
Cook Time: 15 minutes
Total Time: 35 minutes

Protein: 25 grams per serving

YIELD: 4

INGREDIENTS

- sweet potatoes 2 pieces
- 1 bunch of green onions
- Cut 250 g of Haloumi cheese to 1 1/2 x 1/4 inch. slice
- 1/4 cup olive oil
- 2 tablespoons red wine vinegar
- 1 tsp honey
- 2 teaspoons divided smack
- A pinch of salt
- 1/2 teaspoon pepper
- 1 540 mL canned lentils, drain, rinse
- 1/2 radicchio, finely chopped (3 cups)
- 2 cups of parsley leaves

INSTRUCTIONS

1. Preheat to medium barbecue. Soak up 8 skewers of wood in hot tea.
Prick onions, with a fork, all over. Microwave on high plate until mildly tender for 4 min. Let them cool off slightly. Chop the green onion tops thinly and cut the whites into 1-in. sides
2. Cut the potatoes lengthwise into half, then cut into 1/2-in. Sliced slices. Skewers of string cabbage, halloumi and white pieces of green onions, Blend with 1 tbsp of butter.

3. Grill oil. Barbecue skewers, lid closed, tender, about 12 min, rotating every 3 min until grill marks shape and potatoes are crispy.
4. In a small pot, whisk in the remaining butter, vinegar, sugar, 1 tsp sumac, salt, and pepper.
5. Stir in the tops of lentiles, radicchio, parsley and green onion. Sprinkle skewers of remaining sumac.

RED LENTIL COCONUT-MISO SOUP

Active Time: 15 minutes
Cook Time: 20 minutes
Total Time: 35 minutes

Protein: 19 grams per serving

YIELD: 8

INGREDIENTS

- 2 tablespoons of canola oil
- 1 onion, chopped
- 2 carrots peeled and chopped
- 1 1/2 tbsp finely grated raw inger
- 1 900 mL Carton Unsalted Vegetable Soup
- 1 400 mL can coconut milk
- 2 cups of diced butternut squash
- 1 1/4 cup red lentils
- 1 1/2 cup of water, split
- 6 cups of chopped kale, stem removal
- 1/3 cup whiteness o
- 2 tablespoons lemon juice, (optional)

INSTRUCTIONS

1. Heat oil in a medium over large pot. Add carrots and onion, and

simmer for 5 min until softened. Bring the ginger to a boil and simmer until fragrant, 2 min.

2. Add broth, coconut milk, peas, lentils and 1 cup tea. Reduce heat to medium-low and simmer until the lentils and squash begin to break down and thicken the broth, 15 min.

3. Stir in kale, and simmer for 1 min. Whisk miso in a small bowl with remaining 1/2 cup of water until smooth, then whisk in the broth. Take off fire.

4. Stir in lemon juice. For dipping serve with crusty toast

CAULIFLOWER FARRO BOWL

Active Time: 15 minutes
Cook Time: 15 minutes
Total Time: 30 minutes

Protein: 15 grams per serving

YIELD: 4

INGREDIENTS

- 3/4 cup faro
- 1/2 cup green lentils
- 1/2 cup apricot chopped
- 1/3 cup torn mint leaf
- 1/4 cup olive oil
- 1/4 cup tahini
- 2 tablespoons of lemon juice
- 3 tbsp
- 2 garlic pieces, chopped
- 1 teaspoon salt

- 1/4 teaspoon smoked paprika for garnish
- 1 medium cauliflower, cut into small flowers (8 cups)

INSTRUCTIONS

1. Preheat on oven to 400f, then line a parchment baking dish.
2. Bring salted water medium saucepan to a boil. Add farro and lentils, and simmer for 25 to 30 min until tender. Drain well, then pan out. Add apricots, basil, and 2 tbsp of butter, then mix together.
3. Whisk in a medium pot, remaining 2 tbsp of butter, tahini, lemon juice, sugar, garlic, salt and paprika.
4. Arrange cauliflower with half tahini mixture on prepared surface and drizzle, swirling to paint. Roast between bowls until the sides are golden and crispy, 20 to 25 min.
5. Divide farro mix. Cover with cauliflower, cut with remaining tahini and sprinkle with more smoked paprika.

MUSHROOM GRAIN BOWL
Active Time: 15 minutes
Cook Time: 30 minutes
Total Time: 45 minutes

Protein: 22 grams per serving

YIELD: 4

INGREDIENTS
- 500 g sliced mushrooms
- 1/4 cup olive oil
- 3/4 teaspoon salt
- 1/2 red onion, sliced
- 1 garlic, chopped

- Rinse 3/4 cup red and white quinoa
- 1 1/2 cup of water
- 142-g spinach pack, 6 cups
- 540 mL canned lentils, drain, rinse
- 1/2 cup peeled hazelnut, chopped
- 1/3 cup of crushed goat cheese
- 3 tablespoons red wine vinegar

INSTRUCTIONS

1. Preheat oven up to 425f, and line a parchment baking dish.
2. Toss mushrooms on lined baking dish, with 3 tbsp of olive oil and 1/4 tsp salt. Roast the remaining 1 tbsp of oil in a pot over medium until the mushrooms are tender, 20 min. Hot. Attach onion and garlic and cook for around 5 min, stirring until onion is tender.
3. Stir in the quinoa, water and 1/2 tsp of salt left. Boil, then rising flame, covered, to medium-low and simmer for 15 min. Remove from heat and let stand to a wide bowl for 5 min.
4. Transfer; mix with spinach and roasted mushrooms. Apply lentils, hazelnuts, goat cheese, and vinegar to taste.

SQUASH AND PUMPKIN SEED SALAD

Active Time: 15 minutes
Cook Time: 20 minutes
Total Time: 35 minutes

Protein: 17 grams per serving

YIELD: 4

INGREDIENTS

- 1/2 180-g pkg blend of cereal and quinoa, (1/2 cup)

- 400g package of butternut squash prepared, cut into 1 inch. Cube (3 cups)
- 1 coarsely chopped small red onion
- 2 tablespoons olive oil
- 3/4 teaspoon salt
- 1/4 teaspoon pepper
- 3 tablespoons of lemon juice
- 2 cups chopped broccoli florets
- 1 cup of canned focus or Romano beans, drain and rinse
- 1/2 cup dry cherry
- 1/4 cup roasted pumpkin seed
- 1/2 cup crushed sodium reduced feta

INSTRUCTIONS

1. COOK quinoa as guided to box.
2. PREHEAT to 450F. In a baking dish, toss potato, carrot, 1 tbsp of butter, 1/2 tsp of salt, and pepper. Roast halfway through, stirring until fork-tender, 15 to 20 min. Drizzle the lemon juice with 1 tbsp
3. COMBINE quinoa, squash mixture, broccoli, carrots, cherries, pumpkin seeds, 2 tbsp of lemon juice, 1 tbsp of oil left over and 1/4 tsp of salt remaining in a wide cup. Until eating, top off with feta.

PEANUT BUTTER SEED BARS

Active Time: 10 minutes
Cook Time: 10 minutes
Total Time: 20 minutes
Protein: 6 grams per serving

YIELD: 36

INGREDIENTS

- 2 3/4 cup quinoa puff, toast
- 1 cup chopped roast, salted peanuts
- 1/2 cup of white and / or black sesame
- 1/2 cup flaxseed
- 1/2 cup unsalted sunflower seeds
- 1 cup creamy peanut butter
- 2/3 cup honey

INSTRUCTIONS

1. A 9x 13-in cover. Perched baking pan, overhanging on 2 sides In a large bowl Mix quinoa, almonds, sesame seeds, flaxseeds, and sunflower seeds.
2. COMBINE peanut butter and honey over medium in a shallow saucepan, stirring until melted and smooth, 1 until 2 min. Stir in the quinoa mixture until mixed uniformly.
3. Scrape into prepared pan, press tightly into one even layer using a spatula.
4. REFRIGERATE for about 30 minutes, until strong. Cut such into plates. Refrigerate for up to 1 week in a sealed tub, or freeze for up to 3 weeks.

RASPBERRY CHOCOLATE CHIP PROTEIN BARS

Active Time: 10 minutes
Cook Time: 25 minutes
Total Time: 35 minutes

Protein: 6 grams per serving

YIELD: 16

INGREDIENTS

- 1 flaxseed egg, 1 tablespoon flaxseed, 3 tablespoons water
- 1 cup chickpea
- 1 cup mashed banana, about 2 large bananas
- ¾ cup quinoa powder
- ½ cup coconut sugar
- 1 tsp ground cinnamon
- 1/2 teaspoon baking soda
- A pinch of salt
- ¼ cup hemp heart
- ¼ cup frozen raspberry
- 1/4 cup chocolate chip

INSTRUCTIONS

1. Preheat to 350 ° F on burner. Grease and cover a parchment 8x8 baking sheet, then set aside.
2. In a small tub, whisk together the linseed meal and water. Place some 5 minutes aside.
3. When gelled, in a food processor, mix the flax egg, chickpeas, and banana until fully smooth.
4. Attach the dry ingredients (less hemp hearts, chocolate chips, and raspberries) and combine until smooth again. In the remainder of the products pulse.
5. Load the batter into the pan ready for use. If needed, sprinkle with additional chocolate chips and raspberries and bake for 25-30 minutes on the middle rack until a toothpick inserted in the middle comes out clean.
6. Let it cool in the pan for 10-15 minutes, then move to a wire rack and cool before slicing full.

7. Cut into bars 12-16. Place 2-3 days in airtight bag.

APPLE PIE OVERNIGHT QUINOA

Active Time: 5 minutes
Cook Time: 5 minutes
Total Time: 10 minutes

Protein: 6 grams per serving

YIELD: 1

INGREDIENTS

- 1/3 cup quinoa flake
- 2 tablespoons of chia seeds
- 1 tablespoon cannabis
- 1 scoop vegan vanilla protein powder option *
- 1/2 tsp cinnamon
- 1/4 teaspoon ground nutmeg
- 1 cup almond milk + add as needed
- 1 chopped small apple
- 1 tablespoon optional peanut butter

INSTRUCTIONS

In a wide-mouth mason jar, add quinoa, seeds, protein powder, and spices. Add almond milk and mix. Place in refrigerator overnight.

When ready, remove it from the refrigerator, add a little more almond milk if needed, mix and add apples and peanut butter.

HIGH PROTEIN CARROT CAKE CHIA PUDDING

Active Time: 2 minutes
Cook Time: 120 minutes

Total Time: 2 hours 2 minutes

Protein: 6 grams per serving

YIELD: 1

INGREDIENTS

- ¼ Cup quinoa
- ¼ cup grated carrot
- 2 tablespoons of chia seeds
- 2 tablespoons of hemp
- 1/2 tsp cinnamon
- Sea salt pinch
- 1 / 2-3 / 4 cup light coconut milk
- If only 1/2 cup of coconut milk is used, 1/4 cup of water
- Optional add-ins: turmeric medicinal mushrooms, chopped dates, maple syrup, etc.
- Toppings: Grated carrots of sliced bananas, chopped dates, walnuts

INSTRUCTIONS

Add all ingredients to a jar and stir together (minus toppings). Close the lid and place the chia pudding in the refrigerator and set for at least 2 hours (or overnight).

Remove and top with the desired topping. pleasant!

CPSIA information can be obtained
at www.ICGtesting.com
Printed in the USA
BVHW041523191020
591338BV00003B/87

9 781801 095259